Assessing and Treating Emotionally Inexpressive Men

What if your new client, a man in his early 40s, cannot answer basic questions in your initial assessment interview? You were aware that many men do not like to talk about their feelings, but this client seems kind of frozen. You think he might be alexithymic, but you do not know how to assess for that, or even more importantly, how to treat it. *Assessing and Treating Emotionally Inexpressive Men* has answers. Chapters explain why some men are emotionally inexpressive because of their childhood socialization, and the book provides both scales for assessing alexithymia in men and treatment manuals for helping these men became more emotionally self-aware in individual and group therapy. The book also offers case studies that explain how to integrate the authors' approach with any model of psychotherapy. Clinicians will come away from this book with a clear sense of how to treat alexithymia in the early sessions of psychotherapy and thereby improve treatment uptake and outcomes.

Ronald F. Levant, EdD, ABPP, is professor emeritus of psychology at The University of Akron.

Shana Pryor, PhD, is a full-time clinician serving active-duty service members.

The Routledge Series on Counseling and Psychotherapy with Boys and Men

The Routledge Series on Counseling and Psychotherapy with Boys and Men includes books devoted to the process of helping boys and men in counseling and psychotherapy. Topics addressed include: counseling gay boys and men; addictions counseling with boys and men; helping older men; couples counseling with men; counseling gifted boys; assisting men with the transition to fatherhood; helping men with emotional intimacy; counseling boys with attention deficit hyperactivity disorder; counseling boys and men from different racial and ethnic backgrounds; and counseling aggressive boys.

Series Editor: Mark S. Kiselica, Penn State Harrisburg, Pennsylvania, USA

Engaging Men in Couples Therapy
Edited by David S. Shepard and Michelle Harway

Gender in the Therapy Hour
Voices of Female Clinicians Working with Men
Edited by Holly Barlow Sweet

Tough Guys and True Believers
Managing Authoritarian Men in the Psychotherapy Room
John M. Robertson

Men, Addiction, and Intimacy
Strengthening Recovery by Fostering the Emotional Development of Boys and Men
Mark S. Woodford

Breaking Barriers in Counseling Men
Insights and Innovations
Edited by Aaron Rochlen and Fredric E. Rabinowitz

Counseling Widowers
Jason Troyer

Counseling Gay Men, Adolescents, and Boys
A Strengths-Based Guide for Helping Professionals and Educators
Edited by Michael M. Kocet

Religion, Spirituality, and Masculinity
New Insights for Counselors
Anthony Isacco and Jay C. Wade

Assessing and Treating Emotionally Inexpressive Men
Edited by Ronald F. Levant and Shana Pryor

For more information about this series, please visit: https://www.routledge.com/The -Routledge-Series-on-Counseling-and-Psychotherapy-with-Boys-and-Men/book -series/RSCPBM

"Providing psychotherapy for men who 'feel nothing' or deny emotions can prove challenging at best, and often intensely frustrating for many therapists. Long known for his expertise on the special needs of men in psychotherapy, Dr. Ron Levant is joined by Shana Pryor in producing this excellent collection of chapters to guide psychotherapists in assessing and treating emotionally unexpressive men. Packed with clinically validated suggestions for both individual and group work, this book provides both a comprehensive overview and many ideas for starting points with clients who avoid, deny, or fail to recognize many of their own feelings."

Gerry Koocher, PhD, ABPP, former president
of the American Psychological Association

"Augmenting their own considerable expertise, the editors have assembled a remarkable group of scholars and clinicians to produce the definitive volume on this very important and much neglected topic—a must read for any psychotherapist who works with men."

Christopher Kilmartin, PhD, independent
consultant, professor emeritus of psychology,
University of Mary Washington

"Levant and Pryor have given mental health practitioners a true gift. The outstanding contributors in this book have developed a roadmap for treating men who are trying to ditch traditional masculinity and develop loving and fulfilling relationships. The evidence-based research and treatment put forward here belongs on your shelf immediately."

Lenore Walker, EdD, ABPP, professor emerita,
College of Psychology, Nova Southeastern
University

Assessing and Treating Emotionally Inexpressive Men

Edited by
Ronald F. Levant and
Shana Pryor

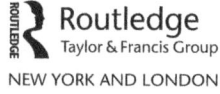

Routledge
Taylor & Francis Group

NEW YORK AND LONDON

Designed cover image: Nuthawut Somsuk © Getty Images

First published 2025
by Routledge
605 Third Avenue, New York, NY 10158

and by Routledge
4 Park Square, Milton Park, Abingdon, Oxon, OX14 4RN

Routledge is an imprint of the Taylor & Francis Group, an informa business

Library of Congress Cataloging-in-Publication Data
Names: Levant, Ronald F, editor. | Pryor, Shana, editor.
Title: Assessing and treating emotionally inexpressive men / edited by Ronald F. Levant and Shana Pryor.
Description: New York, NY : Routledge, 2024. | Series: The Routledge series on counseling and psychotherapy with boys and men | Includes bibliographical references and index. |
Identifiers: LCCN 2024005473 (print) | LCCN 2024005474 (ebook) | ISBN 9781032444697 (paperback) | ISBN 9781032444703 (hardback) | ISBN 9781003378518 (ebook)
Subjects: LCSH: Men--Counseling of. | Men--Mental health. | Emotional maturity in men.
Classification: LCC RC451.4.M45 A87 2024 (print) | LCC RC451.4.M45 (ebook) | DDC 616.89/140811--dc23/eng/20240227
LC record available at https://lccn.loc.gov/2024005473
LC ebook record available at https://lccn.loc.gov/2024005474

ISBN: 9781032444703 (hbk)
ISBN: 9781032444697 (pbk)
ISBN: 9781003378518 (ebk)

DOI: 10.4324/9781003378518

Typeset in Helvetica Neue and Optima
by Deanta Global Publishing, Services, Chennai, India

Contents

Series Editor's Foreword

Mark Kiselica, PhD

Over the course of the past 33 years, I have conducted dozens of workshops on helping troubled boys and men for mental health professionals throughout the United States. One of the most frequently discussed topics raised by the practitioners enrolled in my workshops is the subject of male clients who demonstrate problems with emotional expression. Clinicians regularly reported to me that the men they see in counseling and psychotherapy tend to have trouble putting their feelings into words, feel ashamed about being emotional, and are highly critical of any boy or man who cries. These caring practitioners also noted that these men have difficulty reciprocating the intimate feelings of their partners and children, which is a cause of significant relationship problems in their marital and family relationships. In short, clinical social workers, counselors, marriage and family therapists, psychiatrists, and psychologists recognize that deficits in the emotional makeup of these men have a detrimental impact on the men's lives.

These practitioners are on to something important with their perceptive observations. Although societal stereotypes reflect an overestimation of the emotional difficulties of men (Wester et al., 2002) and many men do in fact have full emotional experiences (Levant et al., 2009), there is evidence that boys who are socialized to be tough and shamed for demonstrating tender feelings are at risk of growing up to be men who adhere to rigid gender roles characterized by restrictive emotionality, which refers to discomfort expressing and experiencing vulnerable emotions (O'Neil, 2008, 2013, 2015). Some of these men suffer with a serious condition referred to as clinical alexithymia, which is characterized by:

> Difficulty identifying feelings, difficulty describing feelings, externally oriented thinking, and a limited imaginal capacity. These characteristics are thought to reflect deficits in the cognitive processing and regulation of emotions and to contribute to the onset or maintenance of several medical and psychiatric disorders (Lumley et al., 2007, p. 230).

However, it is more common for men to be at greater risk than women to struggle with a less severe pattern of restrictive emotionality referred to as Normative Male Alexithymia (Levant et al., 2009). Men who evidence Normative Male Alexithymia (NMA) struggle to put their emotions into words, and they avoid expressing vulnerable emotions, such as fear and sadness, so that they won't appear weak. These emotional deficits appear to have adverse consequences for men and the people in their lives. For example, research findings on Normative Male Alexithymia indicate that NMA is negatively correlated with relationship satisfaction and communication quality and positively correlated with fear of intimacy (Karakis & Levant, 2012). These and other pertinent findings confirm the observations of the clinicians that I had mentioned earlier.

Considering that men with emotional difficulties is a common problem, I realized that producing a book on the topic would be a useful resource for both practitioners and researchers interested in better understanding the phenomenon of emotional inexpressiveness in men, how to assess for it, and how to help men whose lives are hampered by it. As I entertained the idea of adding such a book to the *Routledge Series on Counseling and Psychotherapy with Boys and Men,* I reached out to Dr. Ronald Levant, Professor Emeritus of Psychology at the University of Akron. Dr. Levant is a Fellow and former President of both the American Psychological Association (APA) and the Society for the Psychological Study of Men and Masculinities (SPSMM). A prolific scholar and the author of hundreds of publications and conference presentations, he is one of the world's leading authorities on the psychology of men and masculinities, including the topic of men and their emotions. He cares deeply about men and has dedicated most of his adult life to helping them as a practitioner and a scholar. Long before I started giving workshops on helping boys and men, Dr. Levant noticed troubling emotional deficits in the men he encountered in psychotherapy, so he created interventions designed to help them develop emotional literacy. He also established a systematic line of research focused on studying the emotional development of boys and men and on measuring NMA. He coupled that work with campaigns to raise societal awareness about what happens to those boys and men who are subjected to a harsh socialization process through which they are made to feel ashamed for being sensitive and pressured to be tough and dominant at the cost of true emotional intimacy. Few people have done as much as Dr. Levant to foster gender empathy for men and a scientific approach to studying men's experiences and evaluating a gender-sensitive approach to psychotherapy with men.

A key component of Dr. Levant's many professional activities has been the mentoring of others who share his concern for men, which is how he came to know Ms. Shana Pryor, who is a recent doctorate in counseling psychology from the University of Akron. For the past 10 years, Ms. Pryor has gradually emerged as a rising star and leader among scholars of the psychology of boys, men, and masculinity. She has made numerous contributions to the field, including clinical and research initiatives and peer-reviewed conference presentations and publications that have addressed the impact of trauma on men, patterns of masculinity and compassion, the relationship between masculinity and sexual assault and gun violence, and issues boys experience with discipline, learning disabilities, psychological development, emotions, and discrimination. Much of her important work has involved collaborations with Dr. Levant. When Ms. Pryor was an undergraduate honors student with a major in psychology at Akron, Dr. Levant served as advisor for her honors thesis titled, "What Does Masculinity Have to Do With It? The Correlation Between Sexually Coerced Men and Masculinity." When Ms. Pryor decided to continue with graduate studies in counseling psychology at Akron, Dr. Levant served as advisor for her master's thesis, "Post-Traumatic Growth, PTSD Symptomology, and Shame in Male Survivors of Sexual Trauma: Does Masculinity Play a Role?" One of their most significant collaborations culminated in the publication of their acclaimed book, *The Tough Standard: The Hard Truths About Masculinity and Violence.* In *The Tough Standard*, which was published by Oxford University Press in 2020, Dr. Levant and Ms. Pryor provided a thorough analysis of the link between toxic notions of masculinity and violence while proposing sensible solutions for violence reduction.

I am thrilled that Dr. Levant and Ms. Pryor have decided to combine their impressive talents once again in their production of *Assessing and Treating Emotionally Inexpressive Men*, the latest volume in this book series with Routledge. Drawing from their clinical work with men and cutting-edge research on men and masculinity, including findings from their own empirical investigations, Dr. Levant and Ms. Pryor and their team of contributing scholars have provided a comprehensive resource on how to understand, assess, and treat emotionally inexpressive men in psychotherapy. This book informs practitioners about how a harsh, male socialization process can impair boys and men emotionally and adversely affect their adjustment. The authors offer practical suggestions for assessing NMA in men and helping emotionally inexpressive men to develop the language of emotions and how to express that language in ways that foster their intimate connections with others and an enhanced quality of life. This book also provides scientists with an interest in the psychology of men and masculinity the latest research findings on NMA and how to measure it. Thus, this book is an important addition to the clinical and research literature on the psychology of men. I am deeply grateful to Dr. Levant and Ms. Pryor for this much-needed contribution to the mental health professions and the social science disciplines. I am proud to have their fine work featured in this series.

Mark S. Kiselica, Series Editor
The Routledge Series on Counseling and Psychotherapy with Boys and Men
Penn State Harrisburg
June 20, 2023

REFERENCES

Karakis, E. N., & Levant, R. F. (2012). Is normative male alexithymia associated with relationship satisfaction, fear of intimacy and communication quality among men in relationships? *The Journal of Men's Studies, 20*(3), 179–186. https://doi.org/10.3149/jms.2003.179

Levant, R. F., Hall, R. J., Williams, C. M., & Hasan, N. T. (2009). Gender differences in alexithymia. *Psychology of Men & Masculinity, 10*(3), 190–203. https://doi.org/10.1037/a0015652

Lumley, M. A., Neely, L. C., & Burger, A. J. (2007). The assessment of alexithymia in medical settings: Implications for understanding and treating health problems. *Journal of Personality Assessment, 89*(3), 230–246. doi:10.1080/00223890701629698

O'Neil, J. M. (2008). Summarizing 25 years of research on men's gender role conflict using the gender role conflict scale: New research paradigms and clinical implications. *The Counseling Psychologist, 36*(3), 358–445. https://doi.org/10.1177/0011000008317057

O'Neil, J. M. (2013). Gender role conflict research 30 years later: An evidence-based diagnostic schema to assess boys and men in counseling. *Journal of Counseling and Development, 91*(4), 490–498. https://doi.org/10.1002/j.1556-6676.2013.00122.x

O'Neil, J. M. (2015). *Men's gender role conflict: Psychological costs, consequences, and an agenda for change.* Washington, DC: American Psychological Association. https://doi.org/10.1037/14501-000

Wester, S. R., Vogel, D. L., Pressly, P. K., & Heesacker, M. (2002). Sex differences in emotion: A critical review of the literature and implications for counseling psychology. *The Counseling Psychologist, 30*(4), 630–652. https://doi.org/10.1177/00100002030004008

Foreword

Bruce E. Wampold, PhD

While I was reading *Assessing and Treating Emotionally Inexpressive Men*, I saw an opinion piece in the *Washington Post* that appeared on July 10, 2023, entitled "Men are Lost: Here's a Map Out of the Wilderness," authored by *Post* columnist Christine Emba. Given the topic of Ron Levant's and Shana Pryor's edited book about the challenges encountered by emotionally inexpressive men, I was intrigued to determine the convergences and divergences of an observant, but lay person (Emba), and a psychologically informed perspective (Levant and colleagues).

Emba writes:

> No longer dependent on marriage as a means to financial security or even motherhood (a growing number of women are choosing to create families by themselves, with the help of reproductive technology), women are "increasingly selective," leading to a rise in lonely, single young men – more of whom now live with their parents than a romantic partner ... The data show it, but so does the general mood: Men find themselves lonely, depressed, anxious, and directionless ... Past models of masculinity feel unreachable or socially unacceptable; new ones have yet to crystallize. What are men for in the modern world? What do they look like? Where do they fit? ... Young men everywhere were trying on new identities, many of them ugly, all gesturing toward a *desire to belong* (emphasis added).

Emba goes on to observe how American culture has responded to the "masculinity crisis." On the political right, there are attacks on "woke" culture, which it is claimed has resulted in a collapse of American manhood and masculine strength. On the other hand, Emba notes, enlightened solutions from the progressive side of American culture have a problematic vision as well:

> To the extent that any vision of "nontoxic" masculinity is proposed, it ends up sounding more like stereotypical femininity than anything else: Guys should learn to be more sensitive, quiet and socially apt, seemingly overnight. It's the equivalent of "learn to code!" as a solution for those struggling to adjust to a new economy: simultaneously hectoring, dismissive and jejune.

Emba then goes on to consult with several thought leaders, including Scott Galloway, author, entrepreneur, podcaster, and business school professor, whose focus is on the crisis of single, underachieving young men. To me, as a psychologist, Galloway's response to Embers is particularly uninformative and, more importantly, unactionable:

> My view is that, for masculinity, a decent place to start is garnering the skills and strength that you can advocate for and protect others with. If you're really strong and smart, you will garner enough power, influence, and kindness to begin protecting others. That is it. Full stop. Real men protect other people.

I summarize this opinion piece in some detail to make several points. First, without a doubt, many men in America are distressed, psychologically but also financially, socially, and educationally. Second, the status of men has been politicized, with more rhetoric than solutions. To propose to men an ideal vision of masculinity, from either the right or the left, is ineffective and most likely destructive (or at least not constructive). Third, and most importantly, the absence of reference in this opinion piece to psychology is, from my perspective, a glaring omission. As a corollary to this point, the importance of *emotion* was ignored. Emba's understanding of men's problems could have been greatly enhanced by reading this volume.

The central tenet of *Assessing and Treating Emotionally Inexpressive Men* is that often the core feature of the distress experienced by men is the failure to identify, describe, and express emotions. Emotions are complicated beasts. Like many psychological phenomena, the idea of emotions is recognized by all humans. Ask most humans about the subject and they will have a theory of emotions, describing what they are, why they exist, and what makes them healthy or unhealthy. These theories are referred to as folk psychology. Most everyone would attest to desiring joy and a distaste for fear or disgust. But emotions evolved for a reason – they are critical to survival, as they motivate us to behave in adaptive ways and are critical to managing social relations. Like most evolved human characteristics and processes, emotions can be maladaptive as well as adaptive. And to further complicate matters, the expression of emotions varies considerably across cultures. In this way, this is similar to language – humans evolved to use language, but the languages used in different cultures vary dramatically. Normative ideas about emotions typically are naïve and unhelpful – thus, self-help interventions are of limited utility. And certainly, admonitions and recommendations of politicians, influencers, and digital solutions will not be helpful, and quite likely harmful. Fortunately, there is a somewhat archaic solution – psychotherapy.

Ron Levant has dedicated much of his career to understanding men and emotions. In *Assessing and Treating Emotionally Inexpressive Men*, Dr. Levant and his colleagues cover the entire landscape – theory, evidence, and clinical practice – of the nature of alexithymia and its pernicious effect on men's lives. It is important to keep a central tenet in mind when reading this volume. The information contained in this volume is not intended exclusively for therapists who specialize in working with men, nor does it add another treatment to the overflowing compendium of psychological treatments. The point is that the lives of many are affected by emotionally unexpressive men and therapists should keep this in mind, regardless of the characteristics of the client with whom they are working or the theoretical approach they are using. Alexithymia Reduction Therapy (ART), which is central to this volume, can be integrated with any theoretical orientation.

Let's be clear. This is not a techniques book and readers should not turn to the clinical material on ART without reading the introductory chapters. It is important to understand emotions, men's socialization, and the syndrome of alexithymia, particularly for men, and how emotional inexpressiveness leads to distress and dysfunction (Part I). This material provides a new context for case conceptualization and creates opportunities for therapeutic strategies that may have not come to mind. Part II covers the assessment of alexithymia, presenting scales, how they could be used in practice, and in-depth psychometric validation. Part III describes ART for individual and group modalities, with a strong emphasis on psychoeducation as well as evidence for the efficacy of ART. Finally, Part IV presents case studies of treatment. Clearly, this volume is an integration of science and practice, providing a comprehensive coverage of the topic.

Finally, a few caveats, which are consistent with a careful reading of the clinical material. An understanding of how men's inexpression is problematic should not lead to the conclusion that all men's problems emanate from such emotional issues. Proper assessment is needed (see Part II) as well as a willingness to test clinical conjectures with the client and their response to therapy. A shared understanding and collaborative work are critical in all psychotherapy, but perhaps extremely important when a therapist helps an inexpressive man venture into the (unknown to him) world of emotions. As well, it is vital to understand that there is no universal model for what is healthy emotional experience and expression (see *Between Us: How Cultures Create Emotions*, Batja Mesquita, for example), so as therapists we need to be culturally sensitive to differences in not only expression of emotions but differences in the actual emotions themselves.

Contrasting the approach taken by Dr. Levant and his colleagues with the suggestions in Christine Emba's Washington Post opinion piece makes it clear what psychology, and *Assessing and Treating Emotionally Inexpressive Men* in particular, have to offer in terms of working with men struggling in today's world. Yes, psychotherapy originated as a means to assist an individual client, but when conceptualized as it is in Dr. Levant's volume, it is an intervention to better society, accomplished one client (or one group of clients) at a time. We should recognize and celebrate the power of psychotherapy, for individuals and for society.

Bruce E. Wampold, PhD, ABPP
Professor Emeritus, University of Wisconsin-Madison
Chief Scientist, Skillsetter, Inc.
Chief Clinical Officer, CarePaths, Inc.

Acknowledgments

Chapter 1. The text from the section titled "Origins" through the section titled "Transforming Vulnerable Emotions into Anger," is adapted with permission of the Licensor through PLSclear. Copyright © by Oxford University Press. The official citation that should be used in referencing this material is Levant, R. F., & Pryor, S. (2020). *The tough standard: The hard truths about masculinity and violence*. New York: Oxford University Press. Reproduced with permission of the Licensor through PLSclear.

Chapter 2, Table 1. Copyright © 2006 by the American Psychological Association. Reproduced and adapted with permission. The official citation that should be used in referencing this material is Levant, R. F., Good, G. E., Cook, S., O'Neil, J., Smalley, K. B., Owen, K. A., & Richmond, K. (2006). Validation of the normative male alexithymia scale: Measurement of a gender-linked syndrome. *Psychology of Men and Masculinity, 7*, 212–224. https://doi.org/10.1037/1524-9220.7.4.212 No further reproduction or distribution is permitted without written permission from the American Psychological Association.

Chapter 2, Figure 1. Copyright © 2004 by Iverson M. Eicken, PhD Reproduced with permission.

Chapter 3, entire chapter. Copyright © 2014 by the American Psychological Association. Reproduced and adapted with permission. The official citation that should be used in referencing this material is Levant, R. F., Allen, P. A., & Lien, M.-C. (2014). Alexithymia in men: how and when does the deficit in the processing of emotions occur? *Psychology of Men and Masculinity, 15*,

324–334. https://doi.org/10.1037/a0033860 No further reproduction or distribution is permitted without written permission from the American Psychological Association.

Chapter 4, entire chapter. Copyright © 2022 by the American Psychological Association. Reproduced and adapted with permission. The official citation that should be used in referencing this material is Levant, R. F., Parent, M. C., Ling, S., & Borgogna, N. C. (2022). Variance composition, reliability, validity, and measurement invariance of the Toronto alexithymia scale-20 in nonclinical samples. *Psychology of Men & Masculinities*, *23*(1), 133–142. http://dx.doi.org/10.1037/men0000373 No further reproduction or distribution is permitted without written permission from the American Psychological Association.

Chapter 5, entire chapter. Copyright © 2006 by the American Psychological Association. Reproduced and adapted with permission. The official citation that should be used in referencing this material is Levant, R. F., Good, G. E., Cook, S., O'Neil, J., Smalley, K. B., Owen, K. A., & Richmond, K. (2006). Validation of the normative male alexithymia scale: Measurement of a gender-linked syndrome. *Psychology of Men and Masculinity*, *7*, 212–224. No further reproduction or distribution is permitted without written permission from the American Psychological Association.

Chapter 6, entire chapter. Copyright © 2022 by the American Psychological Association. Reproduced and adapted with permission. The official citation that should be used in referencing this material is Levant, R. F., & Parent, M. C. (2019). The development and evaluation of a brief form of the Normative Male Alexithymia Scale (NMAS-BF). *Journal of Counseling Psychology*, *66*, 224–230. http://dx.doi.org/10.1037/cou0000312 No further reproduction or distribution is permitted without written permission from the American Psychological Association.

Chapters 7 and 8. Alphabetical list of emotion words was reprinted by permission from Rhoda Mills Sommer, LCSW whose website is: https://therapy-ideas.net/wpcontent/uploads/2014/04/feelingwordlist.pdf

Chapter 9, entire chapter. This chapter is adapted with permission from Levant, R. F., Halter, M. J., Hayden, E., & Williams, C. (2009). The efficacy of alexithymia reduction treatment: A pilot study. *Journal of Men's Studies*, *17*(1), 75–84. doi:10.3149/jms.1701.x Reprinted by permission from Sage Publications.

Chapter 10, entire chapter. This chapter is adapted with permission from Levant, R. F. (2000). A quarter century of psychotherapy. In J. Shay & J. Wheelis (Eds.), *Odysseys in psychotherapy* (pp. 187–208). New York: Irvington Press.

Chapter 11, entire chapter. Copyright © 2001 by the American Psychological Association. Reproduced and adapted with permission. The official citation that should be used in referencing this material is Levant, R. F., & Silverstein, L.

(2001). Integrating gender and family systems theories: The "both/and" approach to treating a postmodern couple. In D. Lusterman, S. McDaniel, & C. Philpot (Eds.), *Casebook for integrating family therapy* (pp. 245–252). Washington, DC: American Psychological Association. No further reproduction or distribution is permitted without written permission from the American Psychological Association.

About the Editors

Ronald F. Levant, EdD, ABPP, MBA, DHL (Hon), is a professor emeritus of psychology at The University of Akron. He has developed and evaluated 20 psychological scales designed to assess a variety of gender constructs. These include the Male Role Norms Inventory (MRNI), including the Revised, Short, Very Brief, Adolescent and Adolescent Revised versions, the Normative Male Alexithymia Scale and Brief Form, the Femininity Ideology Scale and Short Form, the Women's Nontraditional Sexuality Questionnaire and Short Form, the Health Behavior Inventory-20 and Short Form, the Fathers' Expectations About Son's Masculinity Scale, the Fathers' Current Expectations About Son's Masculinity Scale, the Reference Group Identity Dependence Scale-Adults-Short Form, the Conformity to Masculine Norms Inventory-30, the Aging Men's Masculinity Ideologies Inventory, and the Duke Health Profile-Brief Form. Dr. Levant's signature contribution has been in establishing the empirical foundation for the "Normative Male Alexithymia" hypothesis. In addition, Levant developed Alexithymia Reduction Treatment (ART), a brief psychoeducational intervention designed to remediate Normative Male Alexithymia in order to prepare men to engage more fully in psychotherapy. ART is designed as an adjunctive treatment that can be administered prior to, or concurrently with, standard care. Further information is at his website: www.DrRonaldLevant.com

Shana Pryor, PhD, is a recent doctorate graduate from the University of Akron. She currently resides in Okinawa, Japan, where she is working with active duty military service members. She has studied Normative Male Alexithymia extensively through the completion of her dissertation on men's emotional in-expression and self-stigma associated with seeking psychological help. She is currently working on projects associated with masculinity and the capacity for compassion. She intends to continue working with military members and hopes to incorporate factors associated with masculinity into her work with clients.

List of Contributors

Phil Allen, PhD, University of Akron

Nicholas C. Borgogna, PhD, Texas Tech University

Stephen W. Cook, PhD, Hardin-Simmons University

Glenn E. Good, PhD, University of Florida

Eric W. Hayden, PhD, BCB, BCN, University of Akron

Margaret Jordan Halter, PhD, Ohio State University

Ronald F. Levant, EdD, ABPP, MBA, DHL (Hon), University of Akron

Mei-Ching Lien, PhD, Oregon State University

Shu Ling, PhD, Cleveland Clinic Akron General Hospital

James M. O'Neil, PhD, University of Connecticut, Storrs, CT

Karen Owen, PhD, Nova Southeastern University

Michael Parent, PhD, MBA, Hope Lab, San Francisco, CA

Shana Pryor, PhD, University of Akron

Kate Richmond, PhD, Muhlenberg College

Louise Silverstein, PhD, Yeshiva University

Bryant Smalley, PhD, PsyD, University of Wyoming

Bruce E. Wampold, PhD, ABPP, University of Wisconsin-Madison

Christine M. Williams, PhD, Independent Practice, Salem, MA

List of Tables and Figures

TABLES

FIGURES

Preface

This book is designed for all mental health clinicians who treat men: psychologists, psychiatrists, psychiatric nurses, social workers, marriage and family therapists, and mental health counselors. It is also intended to serve as a resource for social scientists who may want to investigate the phenomenon of emotionally inexpressive men, by providing a concise compilation of what is known about this topic.

This volume addresses how to understand, assess, and treat emotionally inexpressive men in psychotherapy – that is, men who may suffer from a mild version of alexithymia that has been termed Normative Male Alexithymia.

Alexithymia is a clinical condition in which the client has difficulty in identifying and describing their emotions. The term is composed of Greco-Roman roots: "a" for without, "lexis" for words, and "thymus" for emotions, and literally means "no words for emotions." Sifneos (1973) and Krystal (1982) coined this term to describe the constriction in emotional functioning they observed in their primarily male, psychosomatic patients. While Sifneos (1967) referred to two dimensions – difficulties identifying feelings and difficulties describing feelings, Nemiah et al. (1976) observed that patients with psychosomatic complaints were also preoccupied with the details of external events and objects (termed externally-oriented thinking), and thus included that feature along with the other two in their theoretical definition of alexithymia. Alexithymia so defined was soon observed in patients suffering from other disorders, including eating, substance use, and post-traumatic stress disorders (Taylor, 2004).

Scales have been developed to assess this trait in both clinical and non-clinical populations; the one used most often is the Toronto Alexithymia Scale-20 (TAS-20; Bagby, et al., 1994).

Alexithymic clients are limited in the benefits that they can derive from psychotherapy because all forms of psychotherapy require that clients engage to some degree with their emotional experiences. Even the most behavioral of treatments (e.g., Exposure Therapy) requires that the client identify subtle changes in their anxiety level attendant upon changes in fearful stimuli presented to them. Therefore, treating alexithymia in the early sessions of a course of psychotherapy will likely improve treatment uptake and outcomes for alexithymic clients.

Levant has been working in this area for over three decades. In 1992 he proposed that boys socialized to conform to the masculine norm of restrictive emotionality had an elevated risk of growing up to be men who were at least mildly alexithymic. He subsequently adduced evidence to evaluate that hypothesis. Levant termed this gender-linked form of alexithymia "Normative Male Alexithymia."

The present book covers theory and research on Normative Male Alexithymia, the clinical assessment of men's alexithymia using a general alexithymia scale (Toronto Alexithymia Scale-20), and two versions of a scale developed expressly to tap the gender-linked Normative Male Alexithymia, the Normative Male Alexithymia Scale, and the Normative Male Alexithymia Scale-Brief Form. It also includes treatment. Levant and colleagues developed a manualized treatment for Normative Male Alexithymia in individual and group therapy formats, which was named Alexithymia Reduction Therapy (ART). ART can be integrated into any model of psychotherapy: cognitive behavioral, acceptance and commitment, interpersonal, client-centered, rational emotive, psychodynamic, Adlerian, Gestalt, etc. This book therefore includes updated versions of the ART manuals, including in-session exercises and homework assignments that can be given to clients. We also report on clinical trials assessing ART and provide two clinical case studies illustrating the treatment of alexithymia within the framework of the Bowen Family Theory model.

The present book brings together this corpus of work in an accessible form for mental health clinicians. And it also presents the science involved. As President of the American Psychological Association (APA) in 2005, Levant, reflecting his professional identity as a scientist-practitioner, led the effort to develop the APA Policy on Evidence-Based Practice in Psychology (Goodheart et al., 2006), which was an attempt to resolve the science–practice wars going on in APA at that time. Accordingly, the present book will include (in addition to the focus on practice) several deep dives into the science that supports it, providing reports of the original research that Levant and colleagues conducted. Thus, we have included adaptations of several journal articles and book chapters:

The topic of severity of alexithymia in Chapter 3, the three chapters (4, 5, and 6) on assessment covering the Toronto Alexithymia Scale-20, the Normative Male Alexithymia Scale, and the Normative Male Alexithymia Scale-Brief Form. We have also included a clinical trial of ART in Chapter 9, and the two case studies in Chapters 10 and 11.

It is our hope that this volume contributes in some small way to improving not only men's mental health but also the mental health of people close to them.

REFERENCES

Bagby, R. M., Parker, J. D. A., & Taylor, G. J. (1994). The twenty-item Toronto Alexithymia Scale—I. Item selection and cross-validation of the factor structure. *Journal of Psychosomatic Research, 38*, 23–32. doi:10.1016/0022-3999(94)90005-1

Goodheart, C. D., Levant, R. F., Barlow, D. H., Carter, J., Davidson, K. W., Hagglund, K. J. ... Bullock, M. (2006). Report of the 2005 presidential task force on evidence-based practice. *American Psychologist, 61*, 271–285. https://doi.org/10.1037/0003-066X.61.4.271

Krystal, H. (1982). Alexithymia and the effectiveness of psychoanalytic treatment. *International Journal of Psychotherapy, 9*, 353–378.

Nemiah, J. C., Fryberger, H., & Sifneos, P. E. (1976). Alexithymia: A view of the psychosomatic process. In O. W. Hill (Ed.), *Modern Trends in Psychosomatic Medicine* (Vol. 13, pp. 430–439). London: Butterworths.

Sifneos, P. E. (1967). Clinical observations on some patients suffering from a variety of psychosomatic diseases. *Acta Medicina Psychosomatica, 7*, 1–10.

Sifneos, P. E. (1973). The prevalence of 'alexithymic' characteristics in psychosomatic patients. *Psychotherapy and Psychosomatics, 22*, 255–262. https://doi.org/10.1159/000286529

Taylor, G. J. (2004). Alexithymia: Twenty-five years of theory and research. In I. Nyklicek, L. Temoshok, & A. Vingerhoets (Eds.), *Emotional expression and health: Advances in theory, assessment and clinical applications* (pp. 137–153). New York: Routledge.

PART I

Theory and Research

CHAPTER ONE

The Normative Male Alexithymia Hypothesis[1]

Ronald F. Levant

ORIGINS

I recall when I first became curious about men's emotional inexpressivity. I was on the faculty of Boston University where I directed the Fatherhood Project from 1983–1988. The project offered parental education to fathers, who at the time were noticeably taking on a more involved parenting role than had their predecessors. For example, men were now seen in Harvard Square carrying infants in Snugli baby carriers or pushing strollers.

In an early class, Tim complained about his son standing him up for a father–son hockey game. Not yet aware of the effects of boyhood emotion socialization on some men's ability to give a good account of their emotions, I asked Tim how he *felt* about being stood up. Tim's response was to point his finger and angrily exclaim: "He shouldn't have done it!", not answering my question.

In the Fatherhood Course we used videotaped role-plays to teach fathers parenting skills, in which a father would enact a problematic event, with another father playing the role of the child or another family member. The role-play was videotaped and replayed to analyze the interaction and figure out a better way to handle the situation. In this case, I asked Tim to role-play himself and asked another father to role-play his ex-wife as she delivered the news to him that his son had forgotten the date and gone off with friends, while we videotaped the interaction. I played the video back showing Tim's face falling into a frown and his shoulders slumping. I stopped the tape at that point and asked, "Tim, what were you feeling right then?" Tim, with his right hand rubbing his chin, concentrating intently, said, "I guess I must have felt disappointed."

"'I guess I must have felt disappointed' is the best he can do with this much coaching?," I asked myself. I wondered how a mother in similar circumstance

DOI: 10.4324/9781003378518-2

might react, let's say to her daughter standing her up for a shopping date. I imagined her saying

> Well at first, I was surprised, it's not like her to forget a shopping date. Then I felt angry at being stood up. I was also hurt that she acted with so little regard for my feelings. And I was also worried that that she was perhaps upset with me, and this was her way of letting me know. And I was also disappointed and annoyed – I had planned my day around it and now the day was ruined.

The contrast was striking and caused me to wonder why some men could not give an account of their emotional lives.

GENDER DIFFERENCES IN EMOTION SOCIALIZATION

I had similar experiences with other men who were clients in my part-time psychology practice. Curiosity about these men's difficulties with identifying and describing their emotions drove me to review the research literature in developmental psychology. In my doctoral program at Harvard, I concentrated on child clinical psychology, and as a result knew a bit more about developmental psychology than my classmates.

Focusing on the literature on gender differences in the socialization of emotional expression, I (Levant, 1992, 1998; Levant & Williams, 2009) reviewed the evidence indicating that boys are socialized to restrict the expression of emotions. I observed that boys start life as neonates with greater emotional reactivity and expressiveness than girls; however, a neonate's behavior is limited to crying, eating, eliminating, and sleeping. In addition, boys were found to be more emotionally expressive than girls through 6 months and 1 year of age, when they did much more than cry and sleep, such as coo and gurgle, and direct gestural signals to their mothers (Weinberg, 1992). However, boys became less verbally expressive than girls at about the age of 2 years (Dunn et al., 1987; Fuchs & Thelen, 1988; Haviland & Malatesta, 1981; Malatesta et al., 1989; Schell & Gleason, 1989).

An even larger change happens a few years later. Between the ages of 4 and 6, boys became less facially expressive of emotions than girls. One clever study (Buck, 1977) showed 4-to-6-year-old boys and girls emotionally stimulating slides and videotaped their faces. The child's mother was in an adjacent room watching her own child's face on a television monitor. The researcher's question was: are there differences in mothers' ability to accurately identify the slide shown to her child based on the child's age and gender? At 4 years of age, there were no differences in the accuracy of mothers of sons vs. those of daughters.

But the older the child, the greater the differences, so that by the age of 6 there were significant differences. Mothers of older sons were much less accurate than those of older daughters, indicating that the boys had become much less facially expressive of emotions. So, we must ask: what is happening to children between the ages of 4 and 6? They are in preschool and school, interacting with their peers, who act as gender police for the boys, enforcing conformity to the masculine norm of restrictive emotionality.

The emotional socialization process includes influences from both parents and the child's peers. Mothers manage their more excitable infant boys by dampening their emotional volatility, and fathers begin socializing boys along gender-stereotypical lines as early as age 1 (Haviland & Malatesta, 1981; Lamb, 1977; Lamb et al., 1979; Langlois & Downs, 1980; Siegal, 1987). Parents discourage (and sometimes punish) the expression of vulnerable emotions (such as fear and sadness) in boys, while encouraging this expression in girls (Brody & Hall, 1993; Dunn et al., 1987; Fivush, 1989). This leads boys to suppress, channel, and tune out their vulnerable emotions. In addition, girls' peer group interactions tend to be intimate and to focus on building and maintaining relationships, while boys' groups tend to focus on structured games in larger groups, involving direct competition, teamwork, and toughness (Lever, 1976; Maccoby, 1990; Paley, 1984). Finally, boys who deviate from expectations for emotional reserve often experience harsh punishment by their peers (e.g., Pollack, 1998; Way et al., 2014).

THE NORMATIVE MALE ALEXITHYMIA HYPOTHESIS

Based on this review of the emotion socialization literature, I put forth the "Normative Male Alexithymia hypothesis" (Levant, 1992; Levant & Williams, 2009) – which stated that boys reared to conform to the masculinity norm[2] of restrictive emotionality will likely become at least mildly "alexithymic." The normative nature of alexithymia for boys and men has been observed by others. For example, one of Niobe Way et al's. (2014) teenage research participants put it this way: "It might be nice to be a girl ... then you wouldn't have to be emotionless."

Not All Emotions Are Prohibited

Boys are allowed, even encouraged, to express anger aggressively. And older boys are encouraged by their peers to express lust. In regard to the expression of lust, I can remember as a teenager that a group of boys in our "clubhouse" (which was usually in one boy's garage) would gather around a copy of a magazine like *Playboy* or *Penthouse* and ogle the photos of naked women contained therein.

However, boys reared in homes and neighborhoods that endorse traditional masculinity norms are not allowed to cry nor show fear. That is, they are not allowed to show any kind of emotional vulnerability, which is a rock-bottom requirement of traditional masculinity ideology.

Boys are also restricted from expressing affection or attachment to another person. They cannot be affectionate with another boy lest they be accused of being gay. They cannot express affection to a girl because children play in sex-segregated groups, and boys demonize girls (claiming they had "cooties"). They cannot express affection to their mother lest they be denounced as a "mama's boy." Finally, fathers who subscribe to traditional masculinity norms stop expressing physical affection to their sons around the time they enter school, fearing that they will emasculate them. A magazine story titled "Daddy's Home" illustrated this process:

> Daddy drove into the driveway, parked and got out of the car. His three children were waiting to greet him. He first hugged and kissed one daughter and then another, while his 5-year-old son stood waiting. Daddy said: "No Timmy, men don't do that." Slowly Timmy got reorganized and extended a stiff little manly hand for a handshake.

Transforming Vulnerable Emotions into Anger

Gender role socialization thus teaches boys to lock up their vulnerable and caring emotions. They do this because they have been made to feel enormous shame about even having these emotions. Shame is a powerful emotion. Unlike guilt which is feeling bad over having done a specific action, shame is feeling bad about one's whole self. Fueled by this shame, which in this light can be seen as self-directed hatred, boys learn to transform their vulnerable emotions into anger, aggression, and even rage. Imagine a boy pushed down on the playground by another boy. At some level he probably feels hurt, sad, maybe also afraid. He might even feel betrayed if he thought that boy was his friend. But he knows he must come back up with his fists flying, and certainly not with a face full of tears. So, he takes those vulnerable feelings and transforms them into anger.

Consider for a moment how this works. If someone hurts your feelings, you may feel hurt, sad, and somewhat deflated. But if you shift your focus to the unfairness of what happened – after all you have been very good to this person – the sad feelings can become angry ones. Men who have been socialized in this manner have been known to fly into a rage, igniting much like a match struck to magnesium, when someone hurts their feelings.

ANOTHER PERSPECTIVE: THE KENNEDY–MOORE–WATSON MODEL

Research on men's emotions has been criticized for not sufficiently integrating emotion science (Boise & Hearn, 2017; Wong et al., 2006). In response, Wong and Rochlen (2005) applied the Kennedy–Moore–Watson (KMW) model of emotional expression and inexpression to men's emotional expression, providing important insights into working with men and their emotions. This section summarizes the important work of Wong and colleagues and integrates it with the theory of Normative Male Alexithymia.

The first step of the KMW model is *affective arousal through physiological sensations*. For example, if a man is rejected for a date, he may experience his stomach being in knots, muscle tension, prickly sensations over his skin, or feeling suddenly hot or cold. In this case, the emotion-provoking stimuli (i.e., being turned down for a date) resulted in affective arousal through physiological sensations. However, if the stimulus was not strong enough to elicit a response, he might not experience any bodily sensations at all. In this case, the emotional expression process would never begin.

If he did have physiological arousal, the second step is to *consciously recognize that he is having a bodily response*. Given that some men were socialized as boys to avoid emotional expression, they may not listen to messages their bodies tell them, and as a result may not consciously recognize these feelings. Alternatively, they may choose to ignore them. In either case, the emotional expression process will be disrupted.

However, if he can identify his bodily sensations, the third step is to **label these bodily responses as an emotion**. For example, he might recognize the emotion as disappointment, sadness, or embarrassment. These are vulnerable emotions, so characterized because they make us feel vulnerable. For some men, this step is particularly difficult as they are taught from a young age that vulnerable emotions are associated with femininity, which they are admonished to avoid at all costs. As a result of a disruption at this step, a man's emotional vocabulary may never be fully developed, leading to emotional inexpression.

On the other hand, if signs of physiological arousal are identified as a specific emotion, the man moves onto the fourth step, which is an *evaluation as to whether the identified emotion would be acceptable to express*. Traditional masculinity ideology states that vulnerable and caring emotions (i.e., emotions other than anger) are unacceptable. If the man who was rejected for a date aligns with this belief, he may recognize that he is feeling sad but refuse to express it because to do so is simply not an option. He may therefore choose to either suppress his emotion or display an emotion that is acceptable, anger.

If the man who was rejected does not adhere to traditional masculine norms and is willing to express his sadness and disappointment perhaps to friends or family, he gets to the final stage, which is *considering whether expressing these vulnerable emotions to others would be evaluated positively or negatively*. If the man adheres to traditional masculinity ideology, he will likely view these vulnerable emotions as unacceptable, expecting a negative response (e.g., teasing, minimizing). For some men, it is not uncommon for peers and even family members to react negatively to them when they express vulnerable emotions, often out of their own beliefs about how men should behave. Therefore, it may not be a safe environment for a man who was rejected for expressing his emotions and seeking support, resulting in a lack of emotional expression. If there is an emotionally supportive environment, the rejected individual will be able to seek support and guidance from others around him, reinforcing the idea that expressing his emotions is not only natural but positive.

In this chapter we have summarized the research on the gender differences in emotion socialization, put forth the Normative Male Alexithymia Hypothesis, summarized the important work of Wong and colleagues on the Kennedy–Moore–Watson model and integrated it with the theory of Normative Male Alexithymia. From early in their lives, some men are taught by family, peers, and society to suppress vulnerable emotions for fear of being perceived as unmasculine. As a result, such men are also more likely to turn vulnerable emotions into anger, creating potential damage not only to their relationships but to themselves. Due to this, their self-awareness for bodily sensations that suggest an emotional response is often limited, and the ability to name emotions or obtain an adequate repertoire of emotion words is difficult. An examination of the research and consequences of Normative Male Alexithymia will be provided in the next chapter.

NOTES

1. The text in Chapter 1, from the section titled "Origins" through to the section titled "Transforming Vulnerable Emotions into Anger," is adapted with permission of the Licensor through PLSclear. Copyright © by Oxford University Press. The official citation that should be used in referencing this material is Levant, R. F., & Pryor, S. (2020). *The tough standard: The hard truths about masculinity and violence*. New York: Oxford University Press.
2. And thus the word "normative" in the title of the hypothesis.

REFERENCES

Boise, D. S., & Hearn, J. (2017). Are men getting more emotional? Critical sociological perspectives on men, masculinities and emotions. *The Sociological Review*, 65(4), 779–796. https://doi.org/10.1177/0038026116686500

Brody, L., & Hall, J. (1993). Gender and emotion. In M. Lewis & J. M. Haviland (Eds.), *Handbook of emotions* (pp. 447–460). New York: Guilford.

Buck, R. (1977). Non-verbal communication of affect in preschool children: Relationships with personality and skin conductance. *Journal of Personality and Social Psychology, 35,* 225–236. https://doi.org/10.1037/0022-3514.35.4.225

Dunn, J., Bretherton, I., & Munn, P. (1987). Conversations about feeling states between mothers and their children. *Developmental Psychology, 23,* 132–139. https://doi.org/10.1037/00121649.23.1.132

Fivush, R. (1989). Exploring sex differences in the emotional content of mother child conversations about the past. *Sex Roles, 20,* 675–691. https://doi.org/10.1007/BF00288079

Fuchs, D., & Thelen, M. (1988). Children's expected interpersonal consequences of communicating their affective state and reported likelihood of expression. *Child Development, 59,* 1314–1322.

Haviland, J. J., & Malatesta, C. Z. (1981). The development of sex differences in nonverbal signals: Fallacies, facts, and fantasies. In C. Mayo & N. M. Henly (Eds.), *Gender and non-verbal behavior* (pp. 183–208). New York: Springer-Verlag.

Lamb, M. E. (1977). The development of parental preferences in the first two years of life. *Sex Roles, 3,* 475–497. https://doi.org/10.1007/BF00287413

Lamb, M. E., Owen, M. J., & Chase-Lansdale, L. (1979). The father daughter relationship: Past, present, and future. In C. B. Knopp & M. Kirkpatrick (Eds.), *Becoming female* (pp. 89–112). New York: Plenum.

Langlois, J. H., & Downs, A. C. (1980). Mother, fathers, and peers as socialization agents of sex-typed play behaviors in young children. *Child Development, 51,* 1217–1247. https://doi.org/10.2307/1129566

Levant, R. F. (1992). Toward the reconstruction of masculinity. *Journal of Family Psychology, 5*(3/4), 379–402. https://doi.org/10.1037/0893-3200.5.3-4.379

Levant, R. F. (1998). Desperately seeking language: Understanding, assessing and treating normative male alexithymia. In W. Pollack & R. Levant (Eds.), *New psychotherapy for men* (pp. 35–56). New York: John Wiley & Sons.

Levant, R. F., & Williams, C. (2009). The psychology of men and masculinity. In J. Bray & M. Stanton (Eds.), *The Wiley-Blackwell handbook of family psychology* (pp. 588–599). Oxford, UK: Blackwell Publishing.

Lever, J. (1976). Sex differences in the games children play. *Social Work, 23,* 78–87.

Maccoby, E. E. (1990). Gender and relationships: A developmental account. *American Psychologist, 45,* 513–520. https://doi.org/10.1037/0003-066X.45.4.513

Malatesta, C. Z., Culver, C., Tesman, J., & Shephard, B. (1989). The development of emotion expression during the first two years of life. *Monographs of the Society for Research in Child Development, 50*(1–2, Serial No. 219).

Paley, V. G. (1984). *Boys and girls: Superheroes in the doll corner*. Chicago: University of Chicago Press.

Pollack, W. S. (1998). *Real boys*. New York: Random House.

Schell, A., & Gleason, J. B. (1989). *Gender differences in the acquisition of the vocabulary of emotion*. Paper presented at the annual meeting of the American Association of Applied Linguistics, Washington, DC.

Siegal, M. (1987). Are sons and daughters treated more differently by fathers than by mothers? *Developmental Review, 7*, 183–209. https://doi.org/10.1016/0273 -2297(87)90012-8

Way, N., Cressen, J., Bodian, S., Preston, J., Nelson, J., & Hughes, D. (2014). "It might be nice to be a girl... then you wouldn't have to be emotionless:" Boys' resistance to norms of masculinity during adolescence. *Psychology of Men and Masculinity, 15*, 241–252. https://doi.org/10.1037/a0037262

Weinberg, M. K. (1992). *Sex differences in 6-month-old infants' affect and behavior: Impact on maternal caregiving* (Doctoral dissertation). University of Massachusetts.

Wong, Y. J., Pituch, K. A., & Rochlen, A. B. (2006). Men's restrictive emotionality: An investigation of associations with other emotion-related constructs, anxiety and underlying dimensions. *Psychology of Men and Masculinity, 7*, 113–126. https:// doi.org/10.1037/1524-9220.7.2.113

Wong, Y. J., & Rochlen, A. B. (2005). Demystifying men's emotional behavior: New directions and implications for counseling and research. *Psychology of Men & Masculinity, 6*(1), 62–72. https://doi.org/10.1037/1524-9220.6.1.62

CHAPTER TWO

Research on Normative Male Alexithymia and Related Phenomena

Ronald F. Levant and Shana Pryor

Alexithymia has been investigated frequently in the psychology of men and masculinity studies for several reasons: It is observed more frequently in men; it is linked with the traditional masculine norm and gender role conflict pattern of restrictive emotionality (Levant et al., 2006; O'Neil et al., 2012); and, research on masculinity has repeatedly found that the requirement to restrict emotional expression is a central aspect of masculinity (Brannon, 1976; Good et al., 1994; Levant et al., 1992; Mahalik et al., 2003; O'Neil, 1981; O'Neil et al., 1986).

In this chapter we summarize research that has been conducted on Normative Male Alexithymia, as well as the research into a closely related set of difficulties that men have in managing their emotional lives – namely emotional dysregulation. For the clinician reader, the information in this chapter is important to have confidence that there is sufficient scientific evidence to support the approach that we present in this volume on the assessment and treatment of emotionally inexpressive men. We have taken this approach because we believe that evidence-based practice is the best form of practice.

We begin by considering demographic variations in alexithymia, covering, in turn, the issue of prevalence, sex differences, racial and ethnic differences, and social class differences. We then consider the myriad consequences of Normative Male Alexithymia – for family life, for the workplace, for health, for relationships, for children, for managing stress, and for psychotherapy. Next, we take up recent research on Normative Male Alexithymia. We wrap up by discussing related research on men's emotional difficulties, focusing on emotional dysregulation, the emotional foundation for men's unwillingness to seek help, and the treatment of alexithymia.

DOI: 10.4324/9781003378518-3

DEMOGRAPHIC VARIATIONS

Although alexithymia has been characterized as normally distributed in the general population (Mattila et al., 2010; Parker et al., 2008), it is non-normally distributed due to its low prevalence. The distribution is negatively skewed (i.e., it is skewed to the low end), whereas the skewness for a normal distribution is zero. Furthermore, it is not uniformly distributed throughout the population, affecting men more frequently than women.

Prevalence

One question that often arises is how prevalent is alexithymia in the United States? The short answer is we do not know. All we really know is that it is a low frequency phenomenon, and that men have the condition slightly more often than women. On the other hand, I often ask my audiences to raise their hands if they know a man who cannot identify and describe his emotions, and almost all hands go up. So too, the family therapist and author Terry Real wrote in one of his books, *I Don't Want to Talk About It*: "The psychiatric term for this is alexithymia and psychologist Ron Levant estimates that close to eighty percent of men in our society have a mild to severe form of it." I do not think it is that high and so I wrote to Mr. Real and corrected that statement. But what is needed is a way to measure the prevalence in the United States.

However, the prevalence has been measured in Finland. According to Salminen et al. (1999, p. 75):

> The prevalence of alexithymia and its association with sociodemographic variables were studied in a sample of 1285 subjects representing the general population of Finland ... The prevalence of alexithymia was 13%. Men were alexithymic almost twice (17%) as often as women (10%). Multivariate analysis showed that alexithymia was associated with male gender, advanced age, low educational level, and low socioeconomic status.

Sex Differences

Although alexithymia affects men more often than women, the literature on sex differences is a bit complex. Kiselica and O'Brien (2001) reviewed the literature on sex differences in alexithymia (primarily measured by the Toronto Alexithymia Scale-20) and found that the majority of the studies reported no sex differences. Our literature review (Levant et al., 2006) initially led us to the same conclusion – namely that men were no more likely than women to suffer from alexithymia, but that soon changed.

Levant et al. (2006) narratively reviewed 45 published studies which examined sex differences in alexithymia. The results are summarized in Table 2.1. The finding of no sex differences was especially clear in the subset of studies that studied clinical populations (psychiatric and medical patients). Specifically, two of these studies found that men scored higher than women on a measure of alexithymia, one study found that women scored higher than men, and ten studies found no significant differences. However, the 32 studies using non-clinical samples presented a different picture: 17 of these studies found males met criteria for alexithymia more often than females, one found females met criteria more often than males, and 14 found no differences between males and females. Most of these non-clinical studies were conducted using the relatively healthy and normal population of college students.

Next Levant et al. (2009) performed a meta-analysis of the literature on sex differences in alexithymia (in which the results of numerous studies are statistically aggregated to analyze the average size of the differences). Based on 41 samples they found consistent differences in mean alexithymia scores between women and men, with men having higher scores on alexithymia scales than women. Like the vast majority (78%) of reported psychological sex differences (Hyde, 2005) the effect was small: Hedges' $d = .22$. There were no significant moderator effects for clinical vs. non-clinical populations or alexithymia measure used, although there were relatively few clinical samples, and most studies used the Toronto Alexithymia Scale-20 (TAS-20).

The findings of the literature review and the meta-analysis complemented the review of the emotion socialization literature detailed above, which found that although boys were more emotionally expressive than girls as neonates and retained this advantage until at least 1 year of age, they fell behind girls with respect to verbal expression of emotions by 2 years of age, and facial expression between the ages of 4 to 6 when they entered school.

Ethnic and Racial Differences

Emotional expression varies with culture. For example, I conducted my (RL) psychological practice in the Boston area, where the two largest White ethnic groups were Italian and Irish Americans. Members of both groups tended to be Catholic, and therefore they would tend to mix in Catholic churches and schools. Accordingly, I saw more than a few Irish-Italian marriages for couples therapy in my practice. These two ethnic groups have historically had very different norms for expressing emotion. The Irish norm is the "stiff upper lip" of the United Kingdom – be stoic and do not express strong emotions. On the other hand, the Italian norm is to be very expressive, dramatic even, which is more typical of southern European cultures. Marital stress arises because of the incompatibility of these two sets of norms regulating emotional expression.

TABLE 2.1 Studies Comparing Males and Females on Measures of Alexithymia[1]

Non-clinical	Clinical	Type of Clinical Sample
Males More Alexithymic than Females		
Vingerhoets et al. (1995)[a]	Taylor et al. (1988)[c]	Psychiatric outpatient
Blanchard et al. (1981)[b]	Saarijärvi et al. (1993)[c]	Medical patients referred to psychiatry
Taylor et al. (1985)[c]		
Kirmayer and Robbins (1993)[c]		
Parker, Bagby et al. (1993a)[d]		
Parker, Taylor et al. (1993b)[d]		
Bagby et al. (1994), Study 1[d]		
Taylor et al. (1996)[d]		
Lane et al. (1996)[d]		
Lane et al. (1998)[d]		
Salminen et al. (1999)[d]		
Carpenter and Addis (2000)[d]		
Honkalampi et al. (2000)[d]		
Parker et al. (2001)[d]		
Joukamaa et al (2003)[d]		
Kokkonen et al. (2003)[d]		
Parker et al. (2003)[d]		
Females More Alexithymic than Males		
Pandey et al. (1996)[c]	Haviland et al. (1994)[d]	Substance abuse patients
No Significant Differences Between Male and Females		
Parker et al. (1989)[c]	Millard and Kinsler (1992)[c]	Chronic pain patients
Pasini et al. (1992)[c]	Taylor et al. (1992)[c]	Psychiatric Outpatient
Wise et al. (1992)[c]	Wise et al. (1992)[c]	Psychiatric Outpatient
Joukamaa et al. (1995)[c]	Zeitlin and McNally (1993)[c]	Panic & OCD patients
Cohen et al. (1994)[c]	Cohen et al. (1994)[c]	Somatizing psychiatric patients
Bagby et al. (1994), Study 2[d]	Bach et al. (1994)[c]	Psychiatric Inpatient, Somatic
Todarello et al. (1995)[d]	Bagby et al. (1994)[d]	Psychiatric Outpatient
Bressi et al. (1996)[d]	Todarello et al. (1995)[d]	Psychiatric & hypertensive patients
Dion (1996)[d]	Bressi et al. (1996)[d]	Medical & Psychiatric outpatients
Berenbaum et al. (1998)[d]	Loas et al. (2001)[d]	Addictive Patients
Yelsma et al. (2000)[d]		
Lumley and Sielky (2000)[d]		
Loas et al. (2001)[d]		
Levant et al. (2003)[d]		

(Continued)

14

TABLE 2.1 (Continued)	
Non Clinical Summary:	*Clinical Summary:*
17 Males > Females	2 Males > Females
1 Females > Male	1 Females > Males
14 Non Significant	10 Non Significant

Notes.
[a]Amsterdam Alexithymia Scale (AAS); [b]Beth Israel Hospital Psychosomatic Questionnaire (BIQ); [c]Toronto Alexithymia Scale (26-item TAS); [d]Toronto Alexithymia Scale-20 (20-item TAS-20)

When the Italian partner is upset, they express it loudly and forcefully, volubly as it were. To the Irish partner, this kind of expression would seem to signal the end of the relationship, and they often acted accordingly, i.e., packed a suitcase and retreated to their mother's home. My role as therapist was largely that of a cross-cultural translator.

Several studies have examined the relationship between alexithymia and traditional masculinity ideology (TMI), with a focus on cultural differences based on race and ethnicity. Using a large racially/ethnically diverse sample (40.7% Latino, 35% White, and 24.3% Black), Levant et al. (2003) found a relationship between TMI and alexithymia in men across these races/ethnicities. After controlling for demographic variables, TMI accounted for unique variance in alexithymia in men. A later analysis of the same diverse sample examined the role of race and gender as moderators of the relationship between TMI and alexithymia (Levant & Wong, 2013). While neither race nor gender moderated the relationship between these two variables, the moderating effect of race on the relationship between TMI and alexithymia was strongly affected by gender: TMI was more strongly related to alexithymia for White men than for racial minority men, whereas TMI was more strongly related to alexithymia for racial minority women than for White women.

Finally, Levant et al. (2015) assessed a mediated moderation model of the relationship between the traditional masculine norm of restrictive emotionality (RE) and alexithymia in men. A central theory-driven proposition is that there is a temporal relationship between men's endorsement of TMI beliefs and their subsequent norm conformity behaviors (c.f., Levant & Richmond, 2016). This is based on gender role strain theory, which posits that discrepancy strain arises when a man fails to live up to his own masculinity ideals (Pleck, 1995). Such strain is akin to cognitive dissonance, an unpleasant experience which drives people to behave in a manner consistent with their beliefs. Furthermore, experimental precarious manhood studies show that undermining men's sense of being masculine (i.e., inducing discrepancy strain) results in demonstrations of their conformity to the masculine norm of toughness (Bosson & Vandello, 2011). Several other studies have identified positive links between endorsement of TMI and conformity to masculine norms (reviewed in Gerdes et al., 2017).

Levant et al. (2015) found that conformity to masculine norms mediated the relationship between TMI and alexithymia – specifically, conformity to the masculine norm of emotional control mediated the positive relationship between belief in the traditional masculine norm of restrictive emotionality and alexithymia. In addition, the positive relationship between RE and alexithymia was stronger for Latino men versus men from other racial groups, but weaker for Asian American men versus men from other racial groups. Finally, the RE by race (Latinos vs. others) moderation effect on alexithymia was mediated through its association with emotional control, providing support for a mediated moderation effect.

Social Class Differences

Social class is another cultural dimension. Lorraine Bray (2003) investigated the relationship between traditional masculinity ideology and levels of emotional awareness, comparing college men and women with men and women working in the trades in Canada. This was a PhD dissertation for which I (RL) served as co-supervisor. The Male Role Norms Inventory and the Levels of Emotional Awareness Scale were administered to 372 males and 188 females living in a northern Canadian community. Regression analyses demonstrated that college males' level of endorsement of traditional masculinity ideology predicted their level of emotional awareness, but this relationship did not exist for trades males. For trades males their age and their need for social approval played a greater role in explaining their level of emotional awareness than did their tendency to endorse traditional masculinity ideology. Analyses using MANCOVA found that trades men endorsed traditional male role norms to a greater degree than did college men, and that both trades men and college men endorsed traditional male role norms to a greater degree than did their female counterparts. It was also demonstrated that the level of emotional awareness varied according to the participant's gender but did not vary according to the participant's occupational/social setting (college student/instructor or trades person). Results generally confirmed sex differences in emotional awareness. Outcomes for trades males were unexpected and require further investigation.

CONSEQUENCES OF NORMATIVE MALE ALEXITHYMIA

As a result of Normative Male Alexithymia, some men do not develop a vocabulary for, or are aware of, many of their emotions. They often have great difficulty finding words to describe their emotions, even when they are in obvious distress. Some may even lack an immediate bodily-felt experience of their emotions, and others tend to rely on cognition to logically deduce what they are feeling. And, as we have stated, some men tend to transform their vulnerable emotions into aggression and to respond with aggression when hurt. Consequently, such men lack the emotional skills that might be applied to self-understanding, self-care, emotional empathy, compassion, and richer interactions with others due to their lack of awareness of emotions. Levant also noted that most men experiencing such gender-linked, mild-to-moderate alexithymia did not display the severe symptoms associated with alexithymia, such as a wooden facial expression, an inability to recognize even the physiological components of emotions, and a *pensee operatoire* cognitive style that focuses on the external details of everyday life.

Consequences for Family Life

It is important to note that some men's difficulties with putting words to one's emotions have become increasingly problematic as modern changes in family structures call for men to take on new roles (Levant, 1990). Men are often expected to take on a greater share of nurturing activities with their children, and the demands of two-career families often call for considerable communication skills. Men need the ability to listen actively, express empathy and compassion, and discuss their own feelings. Because the male role socialization process limits development of these abilities, some men are ill-prepared for these roles (Levant & Kopecky, 1995).

Consequences in the Workplace

Furthermore, because of the dramatic changes in the gender composition of the workplace over the past half-century, greater emotional skills are increasingly called for there as well. The Parity Podcast (https://podcasts.apple.com /us/podcast/parity-podcast/id1555981887) discussed how women and men compare on Zenger and Folkman's (2019) list of leadership competencies. They found that women on average rate higher than men on 17 of the 19 core competencies. These data were generated from surveys of over 60,000 people who work in organizations of all sizes. Women and men were close on a lot of the measured competencies, but there was a 3–7% advantage for women when it came to such competencies as taking initiative, resilience, and inspiring and developing others.

Consequences for Health

In addition, alexithymia has been linked to increased physiological reactivity, higher rates of psychosomatic illness, substance abuse, and greater risk for mental disorders (Bach et al., 1994; Cohen et al., 1994; Haviland et al., 1994; Taylor et al., 1992; Porcelli & Taylor, 2018). Perhaps the greater prevalence of alexithymia among men may be an additional risk factor that combines with men's poorer health behaviors to explain men's greater morbidity and mortality as compared to women (Gough & Robertson, 2017).

Consequences for Relationships

Most relationships except for the most superficial ones require some level of self-disclosure; thus Normative Male Alexithymia will negatively impact relation-ships. I received a request from a colleague that illustrates how cut off from intimate others such men can be: "I am writing to ask you for a direction for a woman who has asked me for a book, article, etc. that would help her hus-band understand what she means by emotional intimacy."[2] As another example, one of my clients reported that his wife complained that there wasn't enough intimacy in their relationship. His reaction: "What does she want me to do, rip her clothes off when she steps through the door and make love to her in the foyer?" This client simply could not conceive of intimacy as occurring through conversation. It is therefore not surprising that Normative Male Alexithymia was negatively correlated with relationship satisfaction and communication quality and positively correlated with fear of intimacy in men in heterosexual relation-ships (Karakis & Levant, 2012).

Consequences for Children

Normative Male Alexithymia affects boys as well. A recent survey of more than 1,000 10-to-19-year-olds (Plan International USA, 2018) found that two-thirds of boys reported that society expects them to "hide or suppress their feel-ings when they feel sad or scared" and that they are supposed to "be strong, tough, 'be a man' and 'suck it up.'" As boys reach late adolescence, they tend to disconnect from their emotions and their peers and become very lonely, as Shankar Vedantam has documented on his NPR podcast "Hidden Brain" (Cohen & Vedantam, 2018).

Consequences for Managing Stress

Normative Male Alexithymia has major consequences for managing personal problems. The inability that some men have in identifying their emotions and putting them into words blocks them from utilizing life's most effective means known for dealing with personal problems, ranging from minor hassles to major traumas. We are of course referring to the process of identifying, thinking about, and discussing one's emotional response to a hurtful remark or action with the person who delivered it, or with a third party (friend, family member, religious counselor, or therapist). Having an emotionally honest conversation about a stressful or hurtful situation with another person provides empathy and emotional support and allows the person to put the incident into perspective and figure out a way to handle it. It also provides an opportunity for emotional relief through crying, which – in and of itself – is another one of life's effective means for reducing stress. In this light, punishing boys for crying and instilling in them a deep sense of shame for even wanting to cry must be seen as an incredibly cruel act. After all, we all have tear ducts, irrespective of our gender. Why would males have them if it were unnatural for boys and men to cry? Finally, consider the implications of the shortest sentence in the New Testament: "Jesus wept."

Blocking these avenues off to them, Normative Male Alexithymia predisposes men to deal with personal problems in less constructive ways, which may involve externalizing their problems, as in aggressive and even violent behavior. Other possible harmful responses include substance use to numb oneself out, so that one does not even feel the painful emotions. Porn addiction, sexual compulsions, and gambling addiction can also accomplish this. Finally, not dealing well with stress can lead to stress-related illnesses, and early death. Furthermore, men who learned all too well as boys to transform their vulnerable emotions into aggression will be more prone to act violently when faced with personal problems and hurt feelings.

Consequences for Psychotherapy

Besides interfering with men's ability to express themselves, connect with others, and reduce stress, Normative Male Alexithymia may limit the ability of those men who live with it to fully benefit from psychotherapy. In particular, the inability to identify and express emotional experiences could leave clients without valuable information about their inner psychological experience. Clients without access to their emotions may find that they are less able to affect changes in their thinking, feeling, and behavior. Furthermore, as noted above, even the most behavioral of treatments (e.g., Exposure Therapy) requires that the client identify subtle changes in their anxiety level with changes in fearful stimuli presented to them. There is some empirical support for these ideas. McCallum et al. (2003) found that alexithymia was associated with poorer outcomes in individual and group psychotherapy. Further, Ogrodniczuk et al. (2004) found that alexithymia was associated with the presence of residual symptoms in patients treated for major depression.

RECENT RESEARCH ON NORMATIVE MALE ALEXITHYMIA

Here we discuss dissertation research of student members of APA's division 51, as well as two neuropsychological projects undertaken by Levant and colleagues, one using semantic priming and the other focusing on event related potentials. These latter two projects were concerned with refining the theory of Normative Male Alexithymia. Finally, we discuss Shields' and colleagues' critiques of our and others work on men's emotional inexpressiveness.

Dissertation Research

Several student members of the Society for the Psychological Study of Men and Masculinities, Division 51 of the American Psychological Association, inspired by Levant's work, did their doctoral dissertations on alexithymia in men. For example, Corey Habben examined alexithymia as male emotional detachment (Habben, 1997). Habben's conclusions about men's tendency to distance themselves from their emotions are echoed by many of our points in this book. Simply put, Habben stated that men have a lot to gain by withholding their emotions such as work success, competition, and survival but that this has become "overgeneralized" and therefore bleeds into all areas of their lives. Consequently, they suffer losses in their relationships, mental health, and physical health, resulting in a zero-sum game.

Eicken (2004) examined the potential relationships between emotional intelligence, alexithymia, universal-diverse orientation, and gender role conflict, and assessed whether these relationships are the same for women as they are for men. Eicken concluded that the relationships are sufficiently different for men and women that conceptualizing the genders separately is warranted. Eicken also conceptualized Normative Male Alexithymia a bit differently than we did, focusing on his observation that, among his male patients, there were only two emotions that men could express, namely rage and lust. He developed a diagram to explain it to his patients, which is reproduced in Figure 2.1.

Semantic Priming

In terms of further research on Normative Male Alexithymia, Levant et al. (2014) conducted a semantic priming experiment and found that men with alexithymia showed more errors in lexical decision performance using target emotion words discouraged by masculine norms (e.g., those that expressed vulnerability, such as sadness or fear) compared with men without alexithymia. These results indicated that these men experienced some level of inhibition when encountering words for prohibited emotions, reflecting internal conflict surrounding those words. In addition, men with and without alexithymia did not differ in their

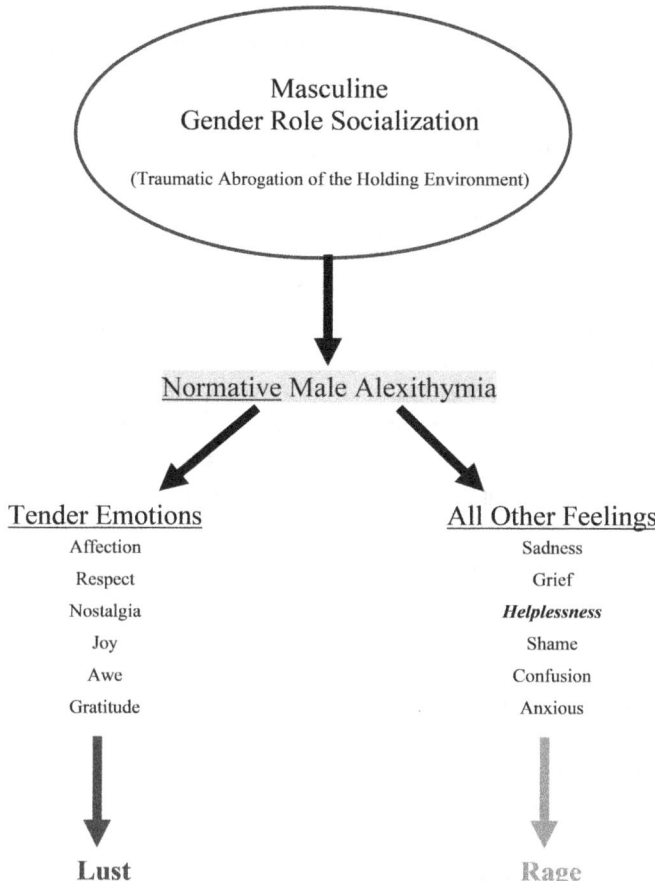

FIGURE 2.1 Eicken's model of Normative Male Alexithymia[2]

accuracy when using target emotion words that are encouraged by masculine norms (e.g., anger).

Event-Related Potentials

Jardin et al. (2019) used event-related potentials (ERPs) to examine the timing of emotional processing in men with and without alexithymia. ERPs measure the changes in voltage in different areas of the brain in relation to sensory, cognitive, or motor events. Compared to traditional behavioral data (e.g., response times), ERPs provide a continuous measure of emotion processing starting from the moment a stimulus is presented. This study used an emotional face discrimination task, in which participants determined the emotion on a face that appeared in the center of the screen. The timing of emotional processing is important because early perceptual inhibition of the participants' reactions to an emotional stimulus would indicate that the psychological defense mechanism of repression caused the alexithymia, suggesting that the men would not have been consciously aware of the emotion conveyed by the face. On the other hand, later cognitive inhibition would indicate that the psychological defense mechanism of suppression caused the alexithymia, suggesting that the men would have been consciously aware of the emotion conveyed by the face.

Using criteria established by the TAS-20 scale developers (Taylor et al., 1988), they tested men, both men who scored high (score > 61), and those who scored low (score < 51), on the TAS-20, on an emotional face discrimination task. The results suggested later processing stages (suppression) as a mechanism for alexithymia in this sample of university students. Furthermore, the results were consistent with Levant's predictions that men would have greater difficulty with vulnerable emotions, such as fear: "Thus, the present results suggest that alexithymic men show greater emotional regulation (specifically inhibition) of a fear response elicited by angry faces (but not the emotional response from happy or neutral faces) relative to controls" (Jardin et al., 2019, p. 11).

Critiques

The psychology of men and masculinity has been critiqued for its conceptualization of men's emotionality (MacArthur & Shields, 2015; Shields, 2013). These researchers asserted that men's purported **rejection of emotions** is not truly present nor valued in the dominant male culture as had been suggested in previous literature (MacArthur & Shields, 2015). A central masculine norm is to avoid anything feminine. In this way, these critics suggest that it is not that men reject emotions, but that they choose not to display emotions that are considered "feminine," but will display "masculine" emotions such as anger. MacArthur and Shields (2015) also highlight exceptions to this rule by pointing to the acceptability of crying by male athletes while playing sports. In this scenario, the men who are crying are doing so in a masculine context (i.e., competing in sports), thereby making a traditionally feminine emotion (i.e., crying) acceptable.

Research that examines sex differences in emotional expression was also critiqued by suggesting that popular culture has influenced scientific writing and vice versa. Shields (2013) proposed that research which utilizes the differences paradigm (e.g., investigation of psychological sex differences by comparing males and females on various psychological attributes, such as emotional expression) transmits essentialist gender messages to popular culture, which in turn influences scientific research. Shields suggested as an antidote that contextual factors should be examined as potential moderators of gender (e.g., observing emotions in context, considering the language of emotion such as gestures), rather than simply examining differences based on sex alone.

Indeed, other research examining sex differences suggests that there is no innate biological difference in emotionality between men and women (Weigard et al., 2021; Wester et al., 2002). Like the suggestions of Shields (2013), Wester and colleagues (2002) stated that sex alone is not enough to explain observed differences in emotional expression. Rather, it is the contextual factors (e.g., relationships, socialization), that need to be examined to avoid appearing to support the essentialist idea that men are inherently less emotional than women.

We agree with these points, as we definitely understand gender to be a social construction that is based on cultural values rather than as determined by biological factors. However, we do believe that the literature on the emotional socialization of children, a literature that we reviewed in Chapter 1, offers an alternative perspective, supporting the idea that gendered social learning shapes emotional expression.

RELATED RESEARCH ON MEN'S EMOTIONAL DIFFICULTIES

Research on men's emotional difficulties has been conducted by a diverse array of researchers from different backgrounds and specialties. It is important to understand men's emotional inexpressiveness not just from the standpoint of alexithymia, but account should also be taken of the various other constructs represented in the research, such as emotion dysregulation as well as the closely associated masculine norms (e.g., Emotional Control and Restrictive Emotionality), and how emotional dysregulation can impact men who have experienced trauma. Finally, we discuss the role of emotion in men's reluctance to seek psychological help, and treatment options.

Emotional Dysregulation

Other research has examined contextual factors in men's *emotional dysregulation*. While emotional dysregulation is different from alexithymia, exploring how men struggle to regulate their emotions may shed some light on men's difficulties with emotion overall. In comparison to women, who are often diagnosed with internalizing disorders (e.g., depression, anxiety), men are more likely than women to be diagnosed with externalizing disorders (e.g., substance use, conduct disorders; Eaton et al., 2012). There is no clear reason as to why this is the case, but research suggests that masculinity may play a role.

In their dynamic model of psychopathology in men, Berke et al. (2018) posited that masculinity is related to psychopathology largely through difficulties with emotion regulation. In other words, men high on some masculinity variables are predicted to struggle with regulating their emotions, which, in turn, predicts psychopathology. It is important to note that it is not correct to say that masculinity ultimately predicts psychopathology; rather, it is more accurate to speculate that there are factors that make developing psychopathology more likely. These factors are contextual in nature and typically build over time – such as gender role socialization, perceived stress associated with performing the masculine role, how much an individual conforms to masculine norms, and interpersonal demands.

The model put forth by Berke and colleagues suggests that these factors operate through a series of inputs, outputs, and outcomes. *Inputs* consist of situations that elicit an emotional response such as being cut off by someone while driving. If the man who was cut-off was taught that a man never lets someone push him around, then this situation may trigger internal masculinity-related cues, influencing how he responds. Let us say that this man was taught by his father to confront anyone who ever challenged him and let us suppose this was reinforced on the playground or at school with him getting into physical fights with other boys. This is where *outputs* come in. Outputs according to this model are physiological, cognitive, and emotional responses to the input in question (i.e., being cut-off). Once the man is cut-off, he experiences physiological responses, perhaps his breath hitches, his muscles tense up, and his heart and respiration rates increase. He may feel angry and may think: "How dare someone cut him off? Who are they to get away with that?" In that moment, the *outcome* part of the model appears. Lost in his anger-fueled thoughts that are brought on by years of masculine socialization and little-to-no emotion regulation abilities, he slams his foot to the gas pedal and begins tailgating the driver who cut him off.

This man was unable to reflect on the fact that he was angry, which might have allowed him to regulate his emotions, by, for example, trying to calm himself down, which in turn caused him to behave in problematic ways. That seems straightforward enough. But how does this lead to psychopathology? Based on the model put forth by Berke and colleagues, the outcome section of the model consists of three parts: short-term, medium-term, and long-term outcomes. The man's response of tailgating someone who cut him off would be classified as a short-term outcome. However, repeat instances of such aggression over time (e.g., fighting at school, displaying aggressive behaviors throughout adulthood) pave the way for medium-term outcomes such as the continuation of distress as he reaps the consequences of his behaviors. These consequences could be isolation and loneliness as he struggles to maintain healthy relationships, the physiological strain that chronic anger has on his body or developing unhealthy coping skills such as alcohol or drug use. If he never learns to regulate his anger in a healthy way, these consequences will build up and become long-term outcomes. For instance, he may become psychologically inflexible and his unhealthy coping strategies like drinking might develop into a substance use disorder. His pattern of aggressive behavior may also develop into some form of conduct disorder or even depression, as depression in some men is typically marked by irritation and aggression (Addis & Hoffman, 2017).

Trauma (Moral Injury)

Our previous example being cut-off while driving illustrates how difficulties in understanding and regulating emotions can occur in everyday life. It is also important to discuss how emotional dysregulation can impact individuals who have a history of experiencing trauma. New research is beginning to examine how emotional dysregulation negatively impacts military veterans who have experienced moral injury (Forkus et al., 2021; Hendrikx & Murphy, 2023). Moral injury can be described as, "perpetrating, failing to prevent, or bearing witness to acts that transgress deeply held moral beliefs and expectations" that "may be deleterious in the long-term, emotionally, psychologically, spiritually, and socially" (Litz et al., 2009, p. 695). Examples of morally injurious events could be the killing of children or non-combatants. A recent study found that potentially morally injurious events (PMIEs) were significantly related to alcohol misuse when there were high levels of negative emotional dysregulation. That is, veterans who experienced PMIEs were at risk of alcohol misuse when they also struggled to regulate their negative emotions. This finding held even after accounting for PTSD symptoms and several demographic variables (i.e., age, race, employment status, relationship status, and branch of service). The same relationship was found for veterans who had difficulty regulating positive emotions as well. In this case, some veterans may have believed that they were undeserving of experiencing positive emotions, or even experienced physiological arousal when feeling positive emotions that could cause trauma-related distress. As a result, such veterans may think of positive emotions as something to be avoided. Regardless of whether the dysregulated emotions were positive or negative in nature, this study suggests that alcohol may be inappropriately used to regulate, avoid, or otherwise cope with emotions.

Emotional Control

Importantly, alcohol misuse in men has also been found to be associated with conforming to the masculine norm of Emotional Control (Gerdes & Levant, 2018). Emotional Control is one of the subscales of the Conformity to Masculine Norms Inventory (CMNI; Mahalik et al., 2003) and captures the tendency for some men to attempt to hold back or contain their emotions (e.g., "I try to keep my emotions hidden"). In a comprehensive review of research of the CMNI subscales,

Gerdes and Levant (2018) reported that men high in Emotional Control were at risk for alcohol use disorder and binge drinking, which, as we have discussed, is also a common way for men to attempt to avoid or otherwise cope with their emotions. On the other hand, men seeking to control their emotions found some benefit in that it helped them control feelings of anger and stress; however, emotional control was also associated with depression, as well as with decreased positive relations with others. Controlling one's emotions was also found to be negatively related to many positive personal traits such as courage, autonomy, resilience, self-esteem, and personal control. This suggests that men may pay a high price for keeping their emotions controlled even if it affords the benefit of preventing them from behaving inappropriately out of stress or anger in the short-term. That is, using fast and easy methods for dealing with one's emotions, such as inhibiting them, does not pan out well in the long run. In addition, men high in Emotional Control may also be less likely to seek psychological health care for depression. Knowing that suicide is considerably higher in men than women (Coleman et al., 2020; Hedegaard et al., 2021), it is especially important for clinicians to be monitoring levels of depression in men who struggle to express or feel their emotions.

As we have seen, it is not enough to say that masculinity, or even emotional dysregulation alone, results in psychopathology. Rather, each person develops their own approach to their world from different life experiences that influence their perception of everyday life situations. This section teaches us that context is important. It is equally not enough to simply examine psychopathology in men without also exploring why they continue to struggle to seek psychological help (Mahalik & Di Bianca, 2021; McDermott et al., 2018; Ramaeker & Petrie, 2019).

The Emotional Foundation for Men's Unwillingness to Seek Help

There is quite a bit of research that examines men's help-seeking attitudes and behaviors (e.g., Berger et al., 2005; Johnson et al., 2012; Levant et al., 2022; Mahalik & Di Bianca, 2021; McDermott et al., 2018; Terlizzi & Zablotsky, 2020). Due to considerations of time and relevancy, we will not be going deeply into this literature. However, it is important to note that men's struggles with their own emotions may be a major factor in why they do not seek help, as research has found that men who strive to control their emotions were not likely to seek psychological services (McDermott et al., 2018; Wong et al., 2017), and had more negative attitudes about seeking psychological help (Mahalik et al., 2003). More recently, there has been research about men's levels of self-stigma about seeking help (i.e., feeling inadequate or bad about oneself for seeking psychological help). This research has found that Emotional Control is associated with self-stigma (Mahalik & DiBianca, 2021).

I (Shana Pryor) recently defended my PhD dissertation on men's self-stigma about seeking psychological help (Pryor, 2023). My study utilized a diverse population consisting of Hispanic/Latino American men, Black/African American men, White/European-American men, and Asian American men. Specifically, I examined how Emotional Control, Normative Male Alexithymia, Disclosure (of one's problems to others), Threatened Masculinity-Related Shame, and Feelings of Inadequacy and Deficiency might be related to men's Self-Stigma. To ascertain whether any relationships between these variables were due to an underlying mental health concern, I also assessed participants' psychological well-being and accounted for it in my final analyses. The results were consistent across all racial/ethnic groups of men. I found that, regardless of one's level of psychological well-being, men who refrained from talking about their feelings or sharing them with others were more likely to struggle to express their emotions and were less likely to disclose their problems to loved ones.

The construct "threatened masculinity-related shame" has only recently been measurable thanks to Gebhard et al.'s (2019) scale development project. This construct posits that men feel shame when they perceive their masculinity is being threatened through such experiences as being called feminine, accused of being gay, or being unable to defend themselves or others. The idea that one's masculinity can be called into question at any time has been referred to as "precarious manhood," which can be summarized in the following statement: "masculinity is hard won and easily lost" (Vandello & Bosson, 2013). Regarding my dissertation research findings, for all men regardless of race/ethnicity, men who worked to control their emotions were less likely to feel threatened masculinity-related shame, suggesting that emotional control could be protective in preventing feelings of shame related to one's perceived lack of masculinity, should it arise. Of course, it may also be that men who control their emotions do not even notice their feelings of shame and would therefore not be able to accurately respond on a self-report scale.

Interestingly, men from all racial/ethnic groups who struggled to express or understand their emotions were more likely to feel threatened masculinity-related shame. On the surface this appears to be a major contradiction as to be relatively unemotional is an honored way of being by traditional masculinity standards. However, consider that suppressing the expression of emotions does not remove the internal experience of the emotions themselves. For men who strive to not express their feelings, and perhaps believe that to feel vulnerable emotions like sadness is tantamount to not being sufficiently masculine, then maybe the internal experience of these emotions is enough to make a man feel as if he is not man enough and to therefore feel shame. There may also be a belief that they are alone in their experiences of emotion and no other man ever feels sad, guilty, or scared, when in fact the opposite is true.

Over all of the racial and ethnic groups that I studied, men who had difficulty expressing and understanding their emotions, and who experienced threatened masculinity-related shame, were more likely to feel inadequate and deficient in general. Importantly, disclosing one's problems to others was also associated with feeling inadequate and deficient. This makes sense as men are taught as boys to never show weakness or vulnerability to others, which also includes talking about their personal struggles. The finding that threatened masculinity-related shame was linked to increased feelings of inadequacy and deficiency is in line with Pleck's (1995) observation that masculinity is unstable in nature (i.e., it is hard won and easily lost). When men do inevitably fail to uphold the demanding standards of masculinity, they feel deep feelings of inadequacy. Finally, I found that men who feel inadequate and deficient were more likely to feel self-stigma about seeking psychological help regardless of race/ethnic group.

Based on my findings, there appears to be important linkages between controlling emotions, having difficulty expressing or understanding one's emotions, and feelings of shame, both in a general sense and related to threats to one's masculinity. These constructs are all connected to feelings of self-stigma and may suggest an explanation for why men who may need psychological help the most are unlikely to seek it.

Treating Alexithymia

Up to this point, we have discussed various psychological perspectives on men's difficulties with emotions. Research has also examined ways in which we might begin treating alexithymia. In a study of adolescents who exhibited violent tendencies, it was found that psychoeducation given in groups reduced alexithymic levels (Bakan et al., 2020).

Further, Neumann et al. (2017) examined the acceptability and initial efficacy of an emotional self-awareness treatment at reducing alexithymia and emotion dysregulation in participants with traumatic brain injury (TBI). I (RL) served as a consultant for this NIH sponsored research project.[3] Seventeen adults with moderate to severe TBI and alexithymia were treated in an outpatient rehabilitation hospital. Eight lessons incorporated psychoeducational information and skill-building exercises teaching emotional vocabulary, labeling, and differentiating self-emotions; interoceptive awareness; and distinguishing emotions from thoughts, actions, and sensations. Thirteen participants completed the treatment. Positive changes were identified for emotional self-awareness and emotion regulation; some changes were maintained several months posttreatment.

Nunes da Silva (2021) also called for the use of psychoeducation in their guidelines for intervention with alexithymic clients. In addition, Nunes da Silva suggested several tenets of intervention which include the assessment of alexithymia, the use of alexithymia in case conceptualization, the importance of emotional awareness and regulation, and the therapeutic alliance. Indeed, for both adults and adolescents, clinicians should create an open dialogue about emotions that encourages exploration and examination into how patients understand, experience, and manage their emotions. In line with previous research discussed in this section, clinicians should also be on the lookout for adverse effects of emotional dysregulation such as substance use, depression, or repeated problematic behaviors in the social, occupational, and personal lives of their clients. Finally, it is important that we assess how men's difficulties with their emotions may influence feelings of shame that may interfere with their ability to seek help.

SUMMARY OF CHAPTER

This chapter aimed to put forth research bearing on Normative Male Alexithymia. While alexithymia is found in people of any sex or gender identity, we have seen that it affects men more frequently, with aspects of masculinity playing key roles in its inception. Indeed, several studies have found links between traditional masculinity ideology, conformity to masculine norms, and alexithymia (Gerdes et al., 2017; Levant et al., 2015). Alexithymic men have also been shown to struggle with recognizing words for emotions that are prohibited by the norms of masculinity – words such as sadness or fear (Levant et al., 2014) – and displayed difficulties identifying their own vulnerable emotions (e.g., fear) resulting from seeing angry facial expressions of others (Jardin et al., 2019).

Most of the studies referenced throughout this chapter were conducted with White/European-American men and it is important to understand if such difficulties in emotional expression are consistent across diverse groups of men. In analyzing cultural differences, we discussed the diverse presentation of emotional expression across cultures. While there are some differences in the expression of emotion such as the contrast between cultures that value dramatic displays of emotion versus those that appear more stoic in their presentation, we found that the relationship between alexithymia and traditional masculinity ideology was present across diverse groups, but with some variations. For instance, the relationship between TMI and alexithymia was present for Latino, White, and Black men, but was stronger for White men than for Latino or Black men (Levant & Wong, 2013). Additionally, the relationship between Restrictive Emotionality and alexithymia was found to be stronger for Latino American men than for Asian American men (Levant et al., 2015). It is clear that masculinity is linked to alexithymia and that this relationship is stable across many racial/ethnic populations.

This chapter also discussed the negative impact of alexithymia on men and those who are close to them. Alexithymia likely results in many negative consequences such as difficulties in family life, the workplace, health, relationships, child development, managing stress, and benefiting from psychotherapy. The masculine socialization process does not encourage boys to be in-tune with their emotions and the emotions of others; *au contraire*, it actively discourages it. Therefore, boys grow up to be men whose lack of emotional understanding translates to being unable to provide adequate communication, empathy, or compassion either for themselves or for others, making relationships and family life difficult to maintain and in some cases dysfunctional. This is becoming increasingly important as women's transition from the home into the workplace has called for men to take on roles outside of traditionally masculine roles, such as that of being a caregiver or homemaker (Levant, 1990). This can be seen as a challenge and an opportunity for fathers to change the trajectory for their sons' development. Indeed, too many young boys continue to feel that they must be disconnected from their emotions to be effective men (Cohen & Vedantam, 2018; Plan International USA, 2018).

The workplace is no different from the home, with many employers expecting greater communication skills which require competence to deal with one's emotions and the emotions of others among their senior executives. Internally, men are susceptible to increased health-related concerns such as mental disorders (Porcelli & Taylor, 2018), especially as men use unhealthy coping mechanisms to deal with their emotions such as substance use, porn viewing, and gambling. This is particularly important for men with emotional regulation difficulties who are at increased risk for externalizing disorders such as conduct problems (Eaton et al., 2012). When trauma is added to the mix, such as with military veterans who have experienced moral injury, a dangerous situation arises as they turn to alcohol to cover over emotions that they do not know how to deal with (Forkus et al., 2021; Hendrikx & Murphy, 2023). To add to the problem, men who struggle with expressing their emotions are more likely to experience shame and higher levels of self-stigma about seeking help (Pryor, 2023), leading them to turn away from treatment. This point is echoed in other research studies which found that men's tendency to control their emotions was related to an unlikeliness to seek psychological help (McDermott et al., 2018; Wong et al., 2017). Until we begin helping boys and men develop healthy emotional skills, their emotional incompetence will continue to put their health, happiness, and the well-being of themselves and their families at risk.

Not only does alexithymia and other emotional difficulties such as dysregulation create negative consequences, so does traditional masculinity ideology. Endorsement of, or conformity to, traditional masculine norms has been linked to a host of difficulties such as reluctance to discuss condom use with partners, fear of intimacy, lower relationship satisfaction, more negative beliefs about the fathers' role, lower paternal participation in child care, negative attitudes toward racial diversity and women's equality, attitudes conducive to sexual harassment, self-reports of sexual aggression, and lower forgiveness of racial discrimination, to name a few (Levant & Richmond, 2007; Gerdes & Levant, 2018; Mahalik et al., 2006). The relationship between masculinity and pathology (Berke et al., 2018) is also something to note as this might help us understand how men develop some mental disorders and why they might be more reluctant than others to seek help. This research points to the idea that, ultimately, if we want to help men, we must make changes in the socialization process so that being a man is no longer at odds with intimacy, communication, and most importantly, emotional competency.

However, as we have seen in this chapter, there are some ideas about men and emotionality that provide openings so that we might begin tackling these problems, for example, the idea that the culture of masculinity may not be about rejecting emotions at all, and that it is a preference, not an inability, to avoid displaying vulnerable emotions (MacArthur & Shields, 2015; Shields, 2013). Indeed, many men develop their own unique version of masculinity. To assume that the problem and the solution is the same across all men ignores the individual differences among men. Research has already determined that psychoeducation is effective for reducing alexithymia and has provided interventions aimed at increasing awareness and regulation of emotion (Bakan et al., 2020; Naumann et al., 2017; Nunes da Silva, 2021). However, there is more work to be done. Going forward, researchers and clinicians will need to come together to determine the full picture of men's difficulties with emotions to determine the best courses of treatment for each unique presentation of masculinity and emotional difficulties. In addition to treatment, we must also begin looking into prevention efforts to interrupt this insidious process before it takes hold.

We have examined many topics and concepts in this chapter. Overall, the research suggests that alexithymia is wide-reaching, highly impactful, and influenced by masculinity constructs and gender socialization across a range of racial and ethnic groups of men. Other concepts such as emotional dysregulation help us understand the complexity of emotion as difficulties can arise in many ways and impact each person differently. Through the use of psychoeducation and other interventions which encourage the understanding and expression of emotion, we can reverse many of the negative outcomes discussed in this chapter. Following this chapter, we will provide a more in-depth description and understanding of the measures used by both researchers and clinicians to assess for alexithymia.

NOTES

1. Table 1. Copyright © 2006 by the American Psychological Association. Reproduced and adapted with permission. The official citation that should be used in referencing this material is Levant, R. F., Good, G. E., Cook, S., O'Neil, J., Smalley, K. B., Owen, K. A., & Richmond, K. (2006). Validation

of the Normative Male Alexithymia Scale: Measurement of a gender-linked syndrome. *Psychology of Men and Masculinity, 7,* 212–224. https://doi .org/10.1037/1524-9220.7.4.212 No further reproduction or distribution is permitted without written permission from the American Psychological Association.

2. Dr. Vic Frazao, personal communication, October 15, 2019.
3. 2012–2016, NIH STTR, "The Emotion Builder: An Intervention to Treat Emotion Deficits After TBI." Dawn Naumann, PhD, PI.

REFERENCES

Addis, M. E., & Hoffman, E. (2017). Men's depression and help-seeking through the lenses of gender. In R. F. Levant & Y. J. Wong (Eds.), *The psychology of men and masculinities* (pp. 171–196). Washington, DC: American Psychological Association. https://doi.org/10.1037/0000023-007

Addis, M. E., & Mahalik, J. R. (2003). Men, masculinity, and the contexts of help-seeking. *American Psychologist, 58,* 5–14. https://doi.org/10.1037/0003-066X .58.1.5

Bach, M., Bach, D., Bohmer, F., & Nutzinger, D. O. (1994). Alexithymia and somatization: Relationship to DSM-III-R diagnoses. *Journal of Psychosomatic Research, 38,* 529–538.

Bagby, R. M., Parker, J. D. A., & Taylor, G. J. (1994). The twenty-item Toronto Alexithymia Scale—I. Item selection and cross-validation of the factor structure. *Journal of Psychosomatic Research, 38,* 23–32. https://doi.org/10.1016/0022 -3999(94)90005-1

Bagby, R. M., Taylor, G. J., & Parker, J. D. A. (1994). The twenty-item Toronto Alexithymia Scale—II. Convergent, discriminant, and concurrent validity. *Journal of Psychosomatic Research, 38,* 33–40. https://doi.org/10.1016/0022 -3999(94)90006-X

Bakan, A. B., Aslan, G., & Aka, P. (2020). An investigation of the effect of the psychoeducation program provided to alexithymic and violent adolescents on the level of alexithymia. *Journal of Child and Adolescent Psychiatric Nursing, 33*(3), 169–179. https://doi.org/10.1111/jcap.12285

Berenbaum, H., Davis, R., & McGrew, J. (1998). Alexithymia and interpretation of hostile-provoking situations. *Psychotherapy and Psychosomatics, 67,* 254–258. https://doi.org/10.1159/000012288

Berger, J. M., Levant, R. F., McMillan, K. K., Kelleher, W., & Sellers, A. (2005). Impact of gender role conflict, traditional masculinity ideology, alexithymia, and age on men's attitudes toward psychological help seeking. *Psychology of Men and Masculinity, 6,* 73–78. https://doi.org/10.1037/1524-9220.6.1.73

Berke, D. S., Reidy, D., & Zeichner, A. (2018). Masculinity, emotion regulation, and psychopathology: A critical review and integrated model. *Clinical Psychology Review, 66,* 106–116. https://doi.org/10.1016/j.cpr.2018.01.004

Blanchard, E. B., Arena, J. G., & Pallmeyer, T. P. (1981). Psychometric properties of a scale to measure alexithymia. *Psychotherapy and Psychosomatics, 35,* 64–71. https://doi.org/10.1159/000287479

Bosson, J. K., & Vandello, J. A. (2011). Precarious manhood and its links to action and aggression. *Current Directions in Psychological Science, 20*, 82–86. https://doi.org/10.1177/0963721411402669

Brannon, R. (1976). The male sex role: Our culture's blueprint for manhood, what it's done for us lately. In D. David & R. Brannon (Eds.), *The forty-nine percent majority: The male sex role* (pp. 14–15, 30–32). Reading, MA: Addison-Wesley.

Bray, L. H. (2003). *Traditional masculinity ideology and normative male alexithymia* (Unpublished doctoral dissertation). University of Alberta.

Bressi, C., Taylor, G., Parker, J., Bressi, S., Brambilla, V., Aguglia, E., et al. (1996). Cross-validation of the 20-item Toronto Alexithymia Scale: An Italian multicenter study. *Journal of Psychosomatic Research, 41*, 551–559. https://doi.org/10.1016/S0022-3999(96)00228-0

Carpenter, K. M., & Addis, M. E. (2000). Alexithymia, gender, and responses to depressive symptoms. *Sex Roles, 43*, 629–644. https://doi.org/10.1023/A:1007100523844

Cohen, K., Auld, F., & Brooker, H. (1994). Is alexithymia related to psychosomatic disorder and somaticizing? *Journal of Psychosomatic Research, 38,* 119–127. https://doi.org/10.1016/0022-3999(94)90085-X

Cohen, R., & Vedantam, S. (2018, March 19). Guys, we have a problem: How American masculinity creates lonely men. *The Hidden Brain*. Retrieved from https://www.npr.org/2018/03/19/594719471/guys-we-have-a-problem-howAmerican-masculinity-creates-lonely-men

Coleman, D., Feigelman, W., & Rosen, Z. (2020). Association of high traditional masculinity and risk of suicide death: Secondary analysis of the add health study. *JAMA Psychiatry, 77*(4), 435–437. doi:10.1001/jamapsychiatry.2019.4702

Dion, K. L. (1996). Ethnolinguistic correlates of alexithymia: Toward a cultural perspective. *Journal of Psychosomatic Research, 41*, 531–539. https://doi.org/10.1016/S0022-3999(96)00295-4

Eaton, N. R., Keyes, K. M., Krueger, R. F., Balsis, S., Skodol, A. E., Markon, K. E., Grant, B. F., & Hasin, D. S. (2012). An invariant dimensional liability model of gender differences in mental disorder prevalence: Evidence from a national sample. *Journal of Abnormal Psychology, 121*(1), 282–288. https://doi.org/10.1037/a0024780

Eicken, I. M. (2004). The relationship of emotional intelligence, alexithymia, and universal-diverse orientation, to gender role conflict. *Dissertation Abstracts International: Section B: The Sciences and Engineering, 64*(9-B), 4665.

Forkus, S. R., & Weiss, N. H. (2021). Examining the relations among moral foundations, potentially morally injurious events, and posttraumatic stress disorder symptoms. *Psychological Trauma: Theory, Research, Practice, and Policy, 13*(4), 403–411. https://doi.org/10.1037/tra0000968

Gebhard, K. T., Cattaneo, L. B., Tangney, J. P., Hargrove, S., & Shor, R. (2019). Threatened masculinity shame-related responses among straight men: Measurement and relationship to aggression. *Psychology of Men & Masculinities, 20*(3), 429–444. http://dx.doi.org/10.1037/men0000177

Gerdes, Z. T., Alto, K. M., Jadaszewski, S., D'Auria, F., & Levant, R. F. (2017). A content analysis of research on masculinity ideologies using all forms of the Male Role Norms Inventory (MRNI). *Psychology of Men & Masculinity, 19*, 584–599. https://doi.org/10.1037/men0000134

Gerdes, Z. T., & Levant, R. (2018). Complex relationships among masculine norms and health/well-being Outcomes: Correlation patterns of the conformity to masculine norms inventory subscales. *American Journal of Men's Health, 12*, 229–240. https://doi.org/10.1177/1557988317745910

Good, G. E., Wallace, D. L., & Borst, T. S. (1994). Masculinity research: A review and critique. *Applied and Preventive Psychology, 3*, 3–14. https://doi.org/10.1016/S0962-1849(05)80104-0

Gough, B., & Robertson, S. (2017). A review of research on men's physical health. In R. F. Levant & Y. J. Wong (Eds.), *The psychology of men and masculinities* (pp. 197–227). Washington, DC: American Psychological Association.

Habben, C. J. (1997). *Male emotional detachment and alexithymia: Prevalence and impact in men's lives and implications for treatment* (Unpublished doctoral dissertation). Wright State University.

Haviland, M. G., Hendryx, M. S., Shaw, D. G., & Henry, J. P. (1994). Alexithymia in women and men hospitalized for psychoactive substance dependence. *Comprehensive Psychiatry, 35*, 124–128. https://doi.org/10.1016/0010-440X(94)90056-N

Hedegaard, H., Curtin, S. C., & Warner, M. (2021). Suicide mortality in the United States, 1999-2019. *NCHS Data Brief, 398*, 1–8.

Hendrikx, L. J., & Murphy, D. (2023). Associations between international trauma questionnaire complex posttraumatic stress disorder symptom clusters and moral injury in a sample of UK treatment-seeking veterans: A network approach. *Psychological Trauma: Theory, Research, Practice, and Policy.* https://dx.doi.org/10.1037/tra0001426

Honkalampi, K., Hintakka, J., Tanskanen, A., Lehtonen, J., & Viinamaki, H. (2000). Depression is strongly associated with alexithymia in the general population. *Journal of Psychosomatic Research, 48*, 98–104. https://doi.org/10.1016/S0022-3999(99)00083-5

Hyde, J. S. (2005). The gender similarities hypothesis. *American Psychologist, 60*(6), 581–592. https://doi.org/10.1037/0003-066X.60.6.581

Jardin, E., Allen, P. A., Levant, R. F., Lien, M-C, McCurdy, E. R., Villalba, A., Mallik, P., Houston, J. R., & Gerdes, Z. T. (2019). Event related brain potentials reveal differences in emotional processing in alexithymia. *Journal of Cognitive Psychology, 31*, 619–633. https://doi.org/10.1080/20445911.2019.1642898

Johnson, J. L., Oliffe, J. L., Kelly, M. T., Galdas, P., & Ogrodniczuk, J. S. (2012). Men's discourses of help-seeking in the context of depression. *Sociology of Health & Illness, 34*(3), 345–361. https://doi.org/10.1111/j.1467-9566.2011.01372.x

Joukamaa, M., Kokkonen, P., Veijola, J., Laksy, K., Karvonen, J. T., Jokelainen, J., et al. (2003). Social situation of expectant mothers and alexithymia 31 years later in their offspring: A prospective study. *Psychosomatic Medicine, 65,* 307–312. https://doi.org/10.1097/01.PSY.0000030389.53353.BC

Joukamaa, M., Sohlman, B., & Lehtinen, V. (1995). The prescription of psychotropic drugs in primary health care. *Acta Psychiatrica Scandinavica, 92,* 359–364. https://doi.org/10.1111/j.1600-0447.1995.tb09597.x

Karakis, E. N., & Levant, R. F. (2012). Is normative male alexithymia associated with relationship satisfaction, fear of intimacy and communication quality among men in heterosexual relationships. *Journal of Men's Studies, 20,* 179–186. https://doi .org/10.3149/jms.2003.179

Kirmayer, L. J., & Robbins, J. M. (1993). Cognitive and social correlates of the Toronto Alexithymia Scale. *Psychosomatics, 34,* 41–52. https://doi.org/10.1016 /S0033-3182(93)71926-X

Kiselica, M. S., & O'Brien, S. (2001, August). Are attachment disorders and alexithymia characteristic of males? In M. S. Kiselica (Chair), *Are males really emotional mummies? What do the data indicate?* Symposium conducted at the Annual Convention of the American Psychological Association, San Francisco, CA.

Kokkonen, P., Veijola, J., Karvonen, J. T., Laksy, K., Jokelainen, J., Jarvelin, M., et al. (2003). Ability to speak at the age of 1 year and alexithymia 30 years later. *Journal of Psychosonatic Research, 54,* 494–495. https://doi.org/10.1016/ S0022-3999(02)00465-8

Lane, R. D., Sechrest, L., & Riedel, R. (1998). Sociodemographic correlates of alexithymia. *Comprehensive Psychiatry, 39,* 377–385. https://doi.org/10.1016/ S0010-440X(98)90051-7

Lane, R. D., Sechrest, L., Reidel, R., Weldon, V., Kaszniak, A., & Schwartz, G. E. (1996). Impaired verbal and nonverbal emotion recognition in alexithymia. *Psychosomatic Medicine, 58,* 203–210. https://doi.org/10.1097/00006842 -199605000-00002

Levant, R. F. (1990). Coping with the new father role. In D. Moore & F. Leafgren (Eds.), *Problem solving strategies and interventions for men in conflict* (pp. 81–94). Alexandria, VA: American Association for Counseling and Development.

Levant, R. F., Allen, P. A., & Lien, M-C. (2014). Alexithymia in men: How and when does the deficit in the processing of emotions occur? *Psychology of Men and Masculinity, 15,* 324–334. https://doi.org/10.1037/a0033860

Levant, R. F., Good, G. E., Cook, S., O'Neil, J., Smalley, K. B., Owen, K. A., & Richmond, K. (2006). Validation of the normative male alexithymia scale: Measurement of a gender-linked syndrome. *Psychology of Men and Masculinity, 7,* 212–224. https://doi.org/10.1037/1524-9220.7.4.212

Levant, R. F., Hall, R. J., Williams, C., & Hasan, N. T. (2009). Gender differences in alexithymia: A meta-analysis. *Psychology of Men and Masculinity, 10,* 190–203. https://doi.org/10.1037/a0015652

Levant, R. F., Hirsch, L., Celentano, E., Cozza, T. Hill, S., MacEachern, M., Marty, N., & Schnedeker, J. (1992). The male role: An investigation of contemporary norms. *Journal of Mental Health Counseling, 14,* 325–337.

Levant, R. F., & Kopecky, G. (1995). *Masculinity reconstructed changing the rules of manhood – at work, in relationship and in family life.* New York: Plume.

Levant, R. F., McCurdy, E. R., Keum, B. T. H., Cox, D. W., Halter, M. J., & Stefanov, D. G. (2022, April 7). Mediation and moderation of the relationship between men's endorsement of traditional masculinity ideology and intentions to seek psychotherapy. *Professional Psychology: Research and Practice, 53*(3), 234–243. http://doi.org/10.1037/pro0000461

Levant, R. F., & Richmond, K. (2007). A review of research on masculinity ideologies using the male role norms inventory. *Journal of Men's Studies, 15,* 130–146. *https://doi.org/10.3149/jms.1502.130*

Levant, R. F., & Richmond, K. (2016). The gender role strain paradigm and masculinity ideologies. In Y. J. Wong & S. R. Wester (Eds.), *APA handbook on men and masculinities* (pp. 23–49). Washington, DC: American Psychological Association.

Levant, R. F., Richmond, K., Majors, R. G., Inclan, J. E., Rossello, J. M., Heesacker, M., et al. (2003). A multicultural investigation of masculinity ideology and alexithymia. *Psychology of Men and Masculinity, 4,* 91–99. https://doi.org/10.1037/1524-9220.4.2.91

Levant, R. F., & Wong, Y. J. (2013). Race and gender as moderators of the relationship between the endorsement of traditional masculinity ideology and alexithymia: an intersectional perspective. *Psychology of Men and Masculinity, 14,* 329–333. https://doi.org/10.1037/a0029551

Levant, R. F., Wong, Y. J., Karakis, E. N., & Welch, M. W. (2015). Moderated mediation of the relationship between the endorsement of restrictive emotionality and alexithymia. *Psychology of Men and Masculinity, 16,* 459–467. https://doi.org/10.3758/s13428-013-0434-y

Litz, B. T., Stein, N., Delaney, E., Lebowitz, L., Nash, W. P., Silva, C., & Maguen, S. (2009). Moral injury and moral repair in war veterans: A preliminary model and intervention strategy. *Clinical Psychology Review, 29*(8), 695–706. https://doi.org/10.1016/j.cpr.2009.07.003

Loas, G., Corcos, M., Stephan, P., Pellet, J., Bizouard, P., & Venisse, J. L. (2001). Factorial structure of the 20-item Toronto Alexithymia Scale confirmatory factorial analysis in nonclinical and clinical samples. *Journal of Psychosomatic Research, 50,* 255–261. https://doi.org/10.1016/S0022-3999(01)00197-0

Lumley, M. A., & Sielky, K. (2000). Alexithymia, gender, and hemispheric functioning. *Comprehensive Psychiatry, 41,* 352–359. https://doi.org/10.1053/comp.2000.9014

MacArthur, H. J., & Shields, S. A. (2015). There's no crying in baseball, or is there? Male athletes, tears, and masculinity in North America. *Emotion Review, 7*(1), 39–46. https://doi.org/10.1177/1754073914544476

Mahalik, J. R., & Di Bianca, M. (2021). Help-seeking for depression as a stigmatized threat to masculinity. *Professional Psychology: Research and Practice, 52*(2), 146–155. https://doi.org/10.1037/pro0000365

Mahalik, J. R., Good, G. E., & Englar-Carlson, M. (2003). Masculinity scripts, presenting concerns and help-seeking: Implications for practice and training. *Professional Psychology: Theory, Research and Practice, 34,* 123–131. https://doi.org/10.1037/0735-7028.34.2.123

Mahalik, J. R., Lagan, H. D., & Morrison, J. A. (2006). Health behaviors and masculinity in Kenyan and U.S. male college students. *Psychology of Men & Masculinity, 7*(4), 191–202.

Mattila, A. K., Keefer, K. V., Taylor, G. J., Joukamaa, M., Jula, A., Parker, J. D. A., & Bagby, R. M. (2010). Taxometric analysis of alexithymia in a general population sample from Finland. *Personality and Individual Differences, 49*, 216–221. https://doi.org/10.1016/j.paid.2010.03.038

McCallum, M., Piper, W. E., Ogrodniczuk, J. S., & Joyce, A. S. (2003). Relationships among psychological mindedness, alexithymia, and outcome in four forms of short-term psychotherapy. *Psychology and Psychotherapy: Theory, Research and Practice, 76,* 133–144. https://doi.org/10.1348/147608303765951177

McDermott, R. C., Smith, P. N., Borgogna, N., Booth, N., Granato, S., & Sevig, T. D. (2018). College students' conformity to masculine role norms and help-seeking intentions for suicidal thoughts. *Psychology of Men & Masculinity, 19*(3), 340–351. https://doi.org/10.1037/men0000107

Millard, R. W., & Kinsler, B. J. (1992). Evaluation of constricted affect in chronic pain: An attempt using the Toronto Alexythymia (SIC) Scale. *Pain, 50*, 287–292. https://doi.org/10.1016/0304-3959(92)90033-8

Neumann, D., Malec, J. F., & Hammond, F. M. (2017). Reductions in alexithymia and emotion dysregulation after training emotional self-awareness following traumatic brain injury: a phase 1 trial. *Journal of Head Trauma Rehabilitation, 32*(5), 286–295. https://doi.org/10.1097/HTR.0000000000000277

Nunes da Silva, A. (2021). Developing emotional skills and the therapeutic alliance in clients with alexithymia: Intervention guidelines. *Psychopathology, 54*(6), 282–290. https://doi.org/10.1159/000519786

Ogrodniczuk, J. S., Piper, W. E., & Joyce, A. S. (2004). Alexithymia as a predictor of residual symptoms in depressed patients who respond to short-term psychotherapy. *American Journal of Psychotherapy, 82*, 469–473.

O'Neil, J. M. (1981). Male sex role conflicts, sexism, and masculinity: Psychological implications for men, women, and the counseling psychologist. *The Counseling Psychologist, 9*(2), 61–79. https://doi.org/10.1177/001100008100900213

O'Neil, J. M., Helms, B., Gable, R., David, L., & Wrightsman, L. (1986). Gender-role conflict scale: College men's fear of femininity. *Sex Roles, 14*(5/6), 335–350. https://doi.org/10.1007/BF00287583

O'Neil, J. M., Wester, S., Vogel, D., & Danforth, L. (2012). Development and evaluation of the Gender Role Conflict Scale Short Form (GRCS-SF). *Psychology of Men and Masculinity, 13*, 199–210. https://doi.org/10.1037/a0025550

Pandey, R., Mandal, M. K., Taylor, G. J., & Parker, J. D. A. (1996). Cross-cultural alexithymia: Development and validation of a Hindi translation of the 20-item Toronto Alexithymia Scale. *Journal of Clinical Psychology, 52*, 173–176. https://doi.org/10.1002/(SICI)1097-4679(199603)52:2<173::AID-JCLP8>3.0.CO;2-V

Parker, J. D. A., Bagby, R. M., Taylor, G. J., Endler, N. S., & Schmitz, P. (1993). Factorial validity of the 20-item Toronto Alexithymia Scale. *European Journal of Personality, 7*, 221–232. Retrieved from ebscohost.com. https://doi.org/10.1002/per.2410070403

Parker, J. D. A., Keefer, K. V., Taylor, G. J., & Bagby, R. M. (2008). Latent structure of the alexithymia construct: A taxometric investigation. *Psychological Assessment*, *20*, 385–396. https://doi.org/10.1037/a0014262

Parker, J. D. A., Taylor, G. J., & Bagby, R. M. (1989). The alexithymia construct: Relationship with sociodemographic variables and intelligence. *Comprehensive Psychiatry*, *30*, 434–441. https://doi.org/10.1016/0010-440X(89)90009-6

Parker, J. D. A., Taylor, G. J., & Bagby, R. M. (1993a). Alexithymia and the recognition of facial expressions of emotion. *Psychotherapy and Psychosomatics, 59*, 197–202. https://doi.org/10.1159/000288664

Parker, J. D. A., Taylor, G. J., & Bagby, R. M. (1993b). Alexithymia and the processing of emotional stimuli: An experimental study. *New Trends in Experimental and Clinical Psychiatry, 9*, 9–14.

Parker, J. D. A., Taylor, G. J., & Bagby, R. M. (2001). The relationship between emotional intelligence and alexithymia. *Personality and Individual Differences, 30*, 107–115. https://doi.org/10.1016/S0191-8869(00)00014-3

Parker, J. A., Taylor, G. J., & Bagby, M. J. (2003). The 20-item Toronto Alexithymia Scale III. Reliability and factorial validity in a community population. *Journal of Psychosomatic Research, 55*, 269–275. https://doi.org/10.1016/S0022-3999(02)00578-0

Pasini, A., Delle Chiaie, D., Seripa, S., & Ciani, N. (1992). Alexithymia as related to sex, age, and educational level: Results of the Toronto Alexithymia Scale in 417 normal subjects. *Comprehensive Psychiatry, 33*, 42–46. https://doi.org/10.1016/0010-440X(92)90078-5

Plan International USA. (2018). *The state of gender equality for U.S. Adolescents*. Retrieved from: https://www.planusa.org/docs/state-of-gender-equality-summary-2018.pdf

Pleck, J. H. (1995). The gender role strain paradigm: An update. In R. F. Levant & W. S. Pollack (Eds.), *A new psychology of men* (pp. 11–32). New York: Basic Books.

Porcelli, P., & Taylor, G. J. (2018). Alexithymia and physical illness: A psychosomatic approach. In O. Luminet, R. M. Bagby, & G. J. Taylor (Eds.), *Alexithymia: Advances in research, theory, and clinical practice* (pp. 105–126). Cambridge University Press. https://doi.org/10.1017/9781108241595.009

Pryor, S. M. (2023). *The problem and the solution: Exploring factors related to masculinity and self-stigma associated with seeking psychological help* (Unpublished doctoral dissertation). The University of Akron.

Ramaeker, J., & Petrie, T. A. (2019). "Man up!": Exploring intersections of sport participation, masculinity, psychological distress, and help-seeking attitudes and intentions. *Psychology of Men & Masculinities, 20*(4), 515–527. https://doi.org/10.1037/men0000198

Saarijärvi, S., Salminen, J. K., Tamminen, T., & Äärelä, E. (1993). Alexithymia in pychiatric consultation-liason patients. *General Hospital Psychiatry, 15*, 330–333. https://doi.org/10.1016/0163-8343(93)90026-K

Salminen, J. K., Saarijärvi, S., Äärelä, E., Toikka, T., & Kauhanen, J. (1999). Prevalence of alexithymia and its association with sociodemographic variables in the general population of Finland. *Journal of Psychosomatic Research, 46*(1), 75–82. https://doi.org/10.1016/S0022-3999(98)00053-1

Shields, S. A. (2013). Gender and emotion: What we think we know, what we need to know, and why it matters. *Psychology of Women Quarterly, 37*(4), 423–435. https://doi.org/10.1177/0361684313502312

Taylor, G. H., Bagby, R. M., Ryan, D. P., Parker, J. D. A., Doody, F. F., & Keefe, P. (1988). Criterion validity of the Toronto Alexithymia Scale. *Psychosomatic Medicine, 50,* 500–509. https://doi.org/10.1097/00006842-198809000-00006

Taylor, G. J., Parker, J. D. A., Bagby, R. M., & Acklin, M. W. (1992). Alexithymia and somatic complaints in psychiatric outpatients. *Journal of Psychosomatic Research, 46,* 417–424. https://doi.org/10.1016/0022-3999(92)90002-J

Terlizzi, E. P., & Zablotsky, B. (2020). *Mental health treatment among adults: United States, 2019* (NCHS Data Brief, No 380). Hyattsville, MD: National Center for Health Statistics.

Todarello, O., Taylor, G. J., Parker, J. D. A., & Fanelli, M. (1995). Alexithymia in essential hypertensive and psychiatric outpatients: A comparative study. *Journal of Psychosomatic Research, 39,* 987–994. https://doi.org/10.1016/0022-3999(95)00506-4

Vandello, J. A., & Bosson, J. K. (2013). Hard won and easily lost: A review and synthesis of theory and research on precarious manhood. *Psychology of Men & Masculinity, 14*(2), 101–113. https://doi.org/10.1037/a0029826

Vingerhoets, A. J. J. M., Van Heck, G. L., Grim, R., & Bermond, B. (1995). Alexithymia: A further exploration of its nomological network. *Psychotherapy and Psychosomatics, 64,* 32–42. https://doi.org/10.1159/000288988

Weigard, A., Loviska, A. M., & Beltz, A. M. (2021). Little evidence for sex or ovarian hormone influences on affective variability. *Scientific Reports, 11*(1), 1–12. https://doi.org/10.1038/s41598-021-00143-7

Wester, S. R., Vogel, D. L., Pressly, P. K., & Heesacker, M. (2002). Sex differences in emotion: A critical review of the literature and implications for counseling psychology. *The Counseling Psychologist, 30*(4), 630–652. https://doi.org/10.1177/00100002030004008

Wise, T. N., Mann, L. S., & Shay, L. (1992). Alexithymia and the five-factor model of personality. *Comprehensive Psychiatry, 3,* 147–151. https://doi.org/10.1016/0010-440X(92)90023-J

Wong, Y. J., Ho, M.-H. R., Wang, S.-Y., & Miller, I. S. K. (2017). Meta-analyses of the relationship between conformity to masculine norms and mental health-related outcomes. *Journal of Counseling Psychology, 64*(1), 80–93. https://doi.org/10.1037/cou0000176

Yelsma, P., Hovestadt, A. J., Anderson, W. T., & Nilsson, J. W. (2000). Family of origin expressiveness: Measurement, meaning, and relationship to alexithymia. *Journal of Marital and Family Therapy, 3,* 353–363. https://doi.org/10.1111/j.1752-0606.2000.tb00304.x

Zeitlin, S. B., & McNally, R. J. (1993). Alexithymia and anxiety sensitivity in panic disorder and obsessive-compulsive disorder. *American Journal of Psychiatry, 150,* 658–660. https://doi.org/10.1176/ajp.150.4.658

Zenger, J., & Folkman, J. (2019, June 25). Research: Women score higher than men in most leadership skills. *Harvard Business Review.* Retrieved from https://hbr.org/2019/06/research-women-score-higher-than-men-in-most-leadership-skills

CHAPTER THREE

Research on the Severity of Normative Male Alexithymia[1]

Ronald F. Levant, Phillip A. Allen, and Mei-Ching Lien

As mentioned in the Preface, the present book includes adaptations of several prior publications, and the present section is the first one of these, covering the topic of severity of alexithymia.

Levant, in his theory of normative male alexithymia, posited that there is a continuum in its severity, corresponding to the severity of the gender role socialization process. The latter ranges from mild, in which boys were simply instructed that the expression of vulnerable and attachment emotions was not appropriate (either in general, or in certain social contexts), to more severe, in which boys were punished for expressing these emotions, to traumatic, in which boys were severely and/or repeatedly punished to the point that they suffered trauma for expressing these emotions. It is further proposed that different psychological defense mechanisms operate at each of these points on this continuum, from suppression for mild socialization, to repression for severe socialization, to dissociation for traumatic socialization.

THE PRESENT STUDY

The literature on alexithymia in men has relied principally on self-report measures and correlational studies. We wanted to extend that psychometric literature using a large self-report sample to determine whether the evidence implies a dissociation, repression, or suppression mechanism for alexithymia in men. Thus, we assessed the extent to which scores on measures of alexithymia and Normative Male Alexithymia can be differentially and uniquely predicted by scores on measures of dissociation, repression, and suppression, to more precisely examine the mechanism for the deficit in emotional processing. However, as is usually the

DOI: 10.4324/9781003378518-4

case in psychology, there is probably no "one-size-fits-all" answer to this question, due to individual differences in personality. Given the non-clinical nature of the participants (college men), we hypothesized that alexithymia will be more strongly predicted by a measure of suppression than by measures of repression and dissociation, since research on gender role conflict suggests that normally functioning men would likely have had milder experiences of masculine socialization than men suffering from psychiatric disorders (O'Neil, 2008).

METHOD

Participants. A total of 258 men from a large, public, Midwestern research university participated in the study. Ages ranged from 18 to 59 years, with a mean of 22.13 (SD = 5.88). The median age was 20, and the modal age was 19. Most participants identified as European American (79.8%), yet 10.5% identified as African-American. Fewer (3.1% or less) identified as Latino/Hispanic, Asian or Asian/American, Middle Eastern, Bi/Multi-Racial, American Indian, or Other. Most participants (96.5%) identified as heterosexual, with 2.3% or less identifying as Gay or Bisexual. Most of the participants indicated that they were either single and dating one person exclusively (33.3%) or single and not dating anyone (36.4%), although 17.1% identified as single and engaged in casual non-exclusive dating, and 14.4% were married, partnered, or engaged. The median self-identified socioeconomic status was middle class. Finally, in terms of religion, most participants (62.4%) identified as Christian, but 21.3% identified as Agnostic or Atheist, and 11.2% as other. Fewer (1.2% or less) identified as Jewish, Muslim, Hindu, Buddhist, or Pagan.

   Procedure. The study was approved by the university IRB. Undergraduate men 18 years and older were solicited from psychology, computer science, and physics courses (the latter two because more men enroll in these courses than in psychology courses) and offered extra credit for their participation in the study. A web-based survey method with a commercially available survey utility was used to collect the psychometric data. The first page of the site reviewed the informed consent information, and participants who agreed to participate clicked "yes," and were taken the survey, which consisted of nine different questionnaires with 189 questions total. Instruments were presented in the order listed below. After participants completed the questionnaires, they received information on how to obtain the results of the study and course credit for their participation.

Measures

Demographic Questionnaire. This questionnaire inquired about sex/gender, race/ethnicity, age, relationship status, sexual orientation, family/household income, SES, and religion.

Normative Male Alexithymia Scale (NMAS). The NMAS (Levant et al., 2006) is a 20-item inventory designed to assess Normative Male Alexithymia (e.g., "I am often confused about what emotion I am feeling"). Participants answered questions about their own experience of emotions using a Likert-type format (1 = *strongly disagree*; 7 = *strongly agree*), with higher scores indicating higher levels of alexithymia. Exploratory and confirmatory factor analyses indicated that the NMAS consisted of a single 20-item factor. Scores on the NMAS displayed evidence of internal consistency (coefficient α = .92) and test–retest reliability (r = .91) over a one to two month period (Levant et al., 2006). In this study, coefficient α = .92.

Toronto Alexithymia Scale (TAS-20). The TAS-20 (Bagby et al., 1994) is the most widely used measure of alexithymia, a construct referring to a cluster of characteristics including difficulty identifying and describing feelings, and externally oriented thinking. Sample items include, "I am often puzzled by sensations in my body," and "I don't know what's going on inside me." Participants rated their agreement with 20 statements ranging from 1 (*strongly disagree*) to 5 (*strongly agree*), with higher scores indicating greater alexithymia. In the present study, the total scale had a coefficient α of .84. Convergent validity has been demonstrated by negative associations with closely related constructs such as psychological mindedness, need-for-cognition, affective orientation, and emotional intelligence (see Taylor, 2004, for a summary).

The NIMH Center for Epidemiologic Studies Depression Scale (CESD). The CESD (Radloff, 1977) was designed for use in studies of the epidemiology of depression. It consisted of 20 items in which participants were asked to indicate how often they felt or acted in the way depicted over the past week, using a four-point Likert-type scale ranging from 0 = *rarely or none of the time (less than 1 day)* to 3 = *most or all of the time (5–7 days)*. A representative item is: "I was bothered by things that usually don't bother me." Higher total scores suggest greater symptoms of depression compared to lower scores. The coefficient α for this study was .79.

The Positive Affect Negative Affect Schedule (PANAS). The PANAS (Watson & Clark, 1994) is a 20-item scale designed to measure two general factors of self-rated affect – Positive Affect (PA) and Negative Affect (NA). Participants were asked to rate to what extent they have experienced a particular emotional state "on the average," using a five-point Likert-type scale, where 1 = *very slightly or not at all* to 5 = *extremely*. Representative items are "Excited" for positive affect and "Distressed" for negative affect. In the present study coefficient α's were .87 for the PA scale and .86 for the NA scale.

Manifest Anxiety Scale (MAS). Bendig (1956) selected the 20 most consistently valid items from the 50-item Taylor Manifest Anxiety Scale (Taylor, 1953) to create the MAS, a measure of trait anxiety. Participants responded to statements about physiological and subjective symptoms of anxiety in a true–false format (e.g., "I feel anxiety about something or someone almost all the time"). Scores range from 0 to 20, with higher scores indicating greater trait anxiety. Bendig (1956) reported coefficient α of .76. In the present study, coefficient α was .89.

Marlow–Crowne Social Desirability Scale (SDS). The 33-item SDS (Crowne & Marlowe, 1960) measures the tendency to respond in socially desirable ways. Participants assessed statements describing socially desirable or undesirable behaviors in a true–false format, for example, "I never hesitate to go out of my way to help someone in trouble." Scores range from 0 to 33, with higher scores indicating greater defensiveness and more socially desirable responding. Crowne and Marlowe (1960) reported a test–retest reliability of .89 and coefficient α of .88. The coefficient α for the present study was .69.

Index of Self-Regulation of Emotion (ISE). The ISE (Mendolia, 2002; Myers & Derakshan, 2004) is based on the MAS and SDS and was used to measure repression. In this study, we followed the procedure of Wong et al. (2006), and calculated participants' ISE scores using the following formula: ISE = 20 − (MAS score − [SDS score × 20/33]). SDS scores were multiplied by 20/33 to equate the total possible score of the SDS with that of the MAS because the SDS has a higher total possible score than the MAS (a score of 33 compared with 20). Scores range from 0 to 40, with higher scores representing higher levels of repression (low levels of self-reported anxiety and high levels of defensiveness). Construct validity has been demonstrated through many studies demonstrating that repressors tend to employ an avoidant style of information processing, repress negative cognitions, dissociate their somatic reactions from their perceptions of distress, and are hypersensitive to anxiety-provoking information (Furnham et al., 2003; Myers & Derakshan, 2004).

Attitudes Towards Emotional Expression Scale (ATEES). The ATEES (Joseph et al., 1994) is a 20-item measure of beliefs and tendencies regarding emotional expression. Participants rated their agreement with statements on a five-point scale ranging from 1 (*disagree very much*) to 5 (*agree very much*). Scores range from 20–80, with higher scores indicating more negative attitudes toward emotional expression. A representative item is: "I think getting emotional is a sign of weakness." Joseph et al. (1994) reported a coefficient α of .90 for the total scale. In the present study, the total scale had a coefficient α of .97. Evidence for convergent validity was provided through reports of associations between the ATEES overall scale and higher levels of depression, a lack of seeking social support (Joseph et al., 1994), and greater ambivalence toward emotional expression (Laghai & Joseph, 2000).

Dissociative Experiences Scale (DES). The DES (Bernstein & Putnam, 1986) is a 28-item measure of dissociation. Participants were asked to rate how frequently they experience specific dissociative symptoms, using an 11-point scale from 0 (*never experiencing*) to 10 (*constantly experiencing*). A representative item is: "Some people have the experience of driving or riding in a car or bus or subway and suddenly realizing that they don't remember what has happened during all or part of the trip." A meta-analysis (Van Ijzendoorn & Schuengel, 1996) found evidence of convergent validity with other measures of dissociation ($d = 1.82$, $N = 5916$), and of predictive validity with dissociative disorders ($d = 1.05$, $N = 1705$), PTSD ($d = .75$, $N = 1099$) and abuse ($d = .52$, $N = 2108$). However, discriminant validity was less well established. In the present study, the coefficient α was .94

RESULTS

Data Screening and Descriptive Statistics

All participants who began the survey completed it, for a completion rate of 100%. The data were thoroughly screened before conducting statistical analyses to ensure the accuracy of the data file. There were missing data as some participants did not respond to every item. No evident patterns of non-response were found by visually inspecting the missing data, which suggested that they were missing at random; hence we replaced missing values using SPSS-17's Linear Trend at Point method. This is a regression-based single imputation method, in which the existing series is regressed on an index variable scaled 1 to n, and missing values are replaced with their predicted values. Descriptive statistics and bivariate correlations of study variables are presented in Table 3.1.

Regression Analyses

We used hierarchical multiple regression analyses to assess the extent to which scores on measures of alexithymia (TAS-20) and normative male alexithymia (NMAS) can be differentially predicted by scores on measures of dissociation (the Dissociative Experiences Scale, DES), repression (the Index of Self-Regulation of Emotion, ISE), and suppression (the Attitudes Toward Emotional Expression Scale, ATEES), in order to investigate by what mechanism the deficits in emotional processing occur. We hypothesized that suppression, a later cognitive regulation effect, will more strongly and uniquely predict alexithymia scores than the earlier effects of either dissociation or repression.

Alexithymia is associated with anhedonia, including both a tendency to experience negative emotions and a diminished capacity to experience positive emotions (Prince & Berenbaum, 1993). Alexithymia is also related to depression (Bagby et al., 1994). Hence we also included measures of these variables, using

TABLE 3.1 Descriptive Statistics and Correlation Coefficients for All Survey Variables

Scale	1	2	3	4	5	6	7	8	9	10
1. TAS-20		.70**	.34**	-.28**	.42**	.22**	-.11	-.24**	.26**	.61**
2. NMAS			.32**	-.30**	.37**	.20**	-.14*	-.23**	.14*	.72**
3. Depression				-.42**	.61**	.48**	-.25**	-.51**	.32**	.34**
4. Pos Affect					-.29**	-.27**	.24**	.33**	-.06	-.25**
5. Neg Affect						-.45**	-.24**	-.48**	.30**	.41**
6. Anxiety							-.13*	-.90**	.23**	.25**
7. Soc Desire								.54**	.12	-.20**
8. Repression									-.24**	-.30**
9. Dissociation										.29**
10. Suppression										
Mean	44.05	3.44	13.29	36.86	18.73	10.70	16.68	19.73	22.59	54.17
SD	10.10	1.03	6.64	6.67	6.34	4.03	3.31	4.76	12.80	11.80
Alpha	.84	.92	.79	.87	.86	.89	.69	–	.94	.87
Score Range	1–100	1–7	0–60	10–50	10–50	0–20	0–33	0–40	0–280	20–80

Note: N = 258 men. TAS-20: Toronto Alexithymia Scale-20; NMAS: Normative Male Alexithymia Scale; Depression: Center for Epidemiologic Studies Depression Scale; Pos Affect and Neg Affect: Positive and Negative Affect subscales (respectively) of the Positive Affect Negative Affect Schedule; Anxiety, Manifest Anxiety Scale; Soc Desire: Marlowe–Crowne Social Desirability Scale; Repression: Index of Self-Regulation of Emotion; Dissociation: the Dissociative Experiences Scale. Suppression: Attitudes Towards Emotional Expression Scale.
* $= p < .05$; ** $= p < .01$.

45

the Positive Affect Negative Affect Schedule (PANAS, which has two subscales, a measure of negative emotions, or affect, NA, and a measure of positive emotions, or affect, PA), and the Center for Epidemiologic Studies Depression Scale (CESD, a measure of depression) as predictors.

The results are shown in Table 3.2. We conducted two analyses, one with alexithymia (TAS-20) as the criterion variable and one with Normative Male Alexithymia (NMAS) as the criterion variable. In Model 1, Step 1, we tested

TABLE 3.2 A Summary of Hierarchical Multiple Regression Analyses on Alexithymia (TAS-20) and Normative Male Alexithymia (NMAS)

Predictor	Beta Coefficients (Standardized)	Significance	Squared Semi-Partial Correlations (Unique Variance)
Model 1 (Criterion = TAS-20):			
Step 1			
Depression	.201	.177	.017
Positive Affect	−.088	.453	.005
Negative Affect	.208	.169	.018
Repression	.075	.608	.002
Dissociation	.150	.155	.019
Step 2			
Depression	.119	.398	.006
Positive Affect	−.067	.544	.003
Negative Affect	.235	.099	.022
Repression	.169	.223	.012
Dissociation	.093	.350	.007
Suppression	.380	.000	.113
Model 2 (Criterion = NMAS):			
Step 1			
Depression	.057	.705	.001
Positive Affect	−.113	.342	.009
Negative Affect	.293	.057	.035
Repression	−.028	.846	.0004
Dissociation	−.032	.759	.0009
Step 2			
Depression	−.088	.450	.003
Positive Affect	−.075	.408	.004
Negative Affect	.339	.005	.047
Repression	.137	.232	.008
Dissociation	−.133	.108	.015
Suppression	.668	.000	.349

Note: Depression: Center for Epidemiologic Studies Depression Scale (CESD); Positive and Negative Affect: PA and NA subscales (respectively) of the Positive Affect Negative Affect Schedule (PANAS); Repression: Index of Self-Regulation of Emotion (ISE); Dissociation: the Dissociative Experiences Scale (DES); Supression: Attitudes Towards Emotional Expression Scale (ATEES).

whether depression (CESD), positive affect (PA), negative affect (NA), repression (ISE), and dissociation (DES) would predict TAS-20 scores. While the model was significant ($F = 3.95$, $p < .003$), none of the beta coefficients were significant. In Step 2, we simply added suppression (ATEES) as the final predictor. The model was significant ($F = 6.16$, $p < .0001$), and the increment in R-squared was .113 ($F = 14.02$, $p < .0001$). Furthermore, the only significant predictor was suppression, and its squared semi-partial correlation, reflecting the unique variance, was .113. Thus, even when suppression was forced to be entered last, it still was the only significant predictor. This suggests that suppression predicted TAS-20 scores independently of all the other variables.

In Model 2, Step 1, we tested whether depression (CESD), positive affect (PA), negative affect (NA), repression (ISE), and dissociation (DES) predicted normative male alexithymia (NMAS). As in Model 1, Step 1 was significant ($F = 3.58$, $p < .005$), but none of the beta coefficients were significant. In Step 2, we added suppression (ATEES) to the other five predictors. The second step was significant ($F = 15.59$, $p < .0001$), and the increment in R-squared was .349 ($F = 62.98$, $p < .0001$). Both negative affect and suppression were significant predictors. Their squared semi-partial correlations, reflecting unique variance, were .047 and .349, respectively. The results from Model 2 suggested that suppression predicted NMAS scores independently of most of the other variables, with the exception of negative affect, although it accounted for almost three times as much unique variance as negative affect.

DISCUSSION

Summary of Results

Although we theorized that normative male alexithymia and alexithymia could be associated with dissociation, repression, or suppression, given the non-clinical nature of the participants (college men), we hypothesized that they would be more strongly predicted by a measure of suppression than by measures of repression and dissociation, since normally functioning men would likely have had milder experiences of masculine socialization.

The results showed that suppression was a better predictor of alexithymia than were either dissociation or repression, while controlling for positive and negative affect and depression, although both suppression and negative affect predicted Normative Male Alexithymia. However, the squared semi-partial correlations (reflecting unique variance) were substantially larger for suppression than for the other predictors for both alexithymia and normative male alexithymia. Consequently, these regression results provide evidence that suppression is the best predictor of alexithymia and Normative Male Alexithymia in a sample of college men. This is consistent with prior survey research on "restrictive emotionality," a form of men's gender role conflict that is similar to Normative Male Alexithymia (O'Neil, 2008). Wong et al. (2006) found, using regression analyses, that suppression, as measured by the ATEES, was found to be most closely associated with a set of emotion-related variables with restrictive emotionality.

Thus, converging lines of evidence, arising from survey data analyzed by regression techniques (the present study, Wong et al., 2006), to experimental data using semantic priming (as in Levant et al., 2014; Suslow & Junghanns, 2002), implicate suppression as the mechanism for alexithymia and Normative Male Alexithymia. In other words, alexithymic men quell their emotions, but they do experience them. One important implication for theory development is that Gender Role Strain Paradigm theorists (Levant, 2011; Pleck, 1981, 1995; Pollack, 1998), who have characterized the emotional socialization process that occurs during boyhood as "trauma strain," may have overestimated the damaging effects of the male emotional socialization process for most men. Suppression is considered a higher level, less reality-distorting defense mechanism than either repression or dissociation. However, as was previously noted, there is probably no "one size fits all" answer to the question of where the disruption in emotion processing occurs. It is conceivable that repression and dissociation might play stronger roles in community, or, more likely, clinical samples.

LIMITATIONS AND SUGGESTIONS FOR FUTURE RESEARCH

We wish to acknowledge some limitations of the current study which at present may also place some boundaries around the generalizations of results. First, the majority of college men who participated in the investigation were young, European American, heterosexual, and Christian, raising concerns about the generalizability of our findings. Future research should attempt to replicate the present findings with a more diverse population in terms of age, race/ethnicity, sexual orientation, and religion. Moreover, in terms of further investigating the role of repression, dissociation, it would be important to include clinical samples in future research.

Second, as noted above, there are limitations with regard to the present study, which include a potential order-effect in the presentation of the scales, participant fatigue, item similarity between the alexithymia, Normative Male Alexithymia, and suppression measures, low alpha for one scale, the possibility of bias due to socially desirable responding, and the correlational nature of the data. Future research should address these issues.

NOTE

1. Chapter 3, entire chapter. Copyright © 2014 by the American Psychological Association. Reproduced and adapted with permission. The official citation that should be used in referencing this material is Levant, R. F., Allen, P. A., & Lien, M-C. (2014) Alexithymia in men: How and when does the deficit in the processing of emotions occur? *Psychology of Men and Masculinity, 15,* 324–334. https://doi.org/10.1037/a0033860 No further reproduction or distribution is permitted without written permission from the American Psychological Association.

REFERENCES

Bach, M., Bach, D., Bohmer, F., & Nutzinger, D. O. (1994). Alexithymia and somatization: Relationship to DSM-III-R diagnoses. *Journal of Psychosomatic Research, 38,* 529–538.

Bagby, R. M., Parker, J. D. A., & Taylor, G. J. (1994). The twenty-item Toronto Alexithymia Scale—I. Item selection and cross-validation of the factor structure. *Journal of Psychosomatic Research, 38,* 23–32. https://doi.org/10.1016/0022 -3999(94)90005-1

Bagby, R. M., Taylor, G. J., & Parker, J. D. A. (1994). The twenty-item Toronto Alexithymia Scale--II. Convergent, discriminant, and concurrent validity. *Journal of Psychosomatic Research, 38,* 33–40. https://doi.org/10.1016/0022 -3999(94)90006-X

Bakan, A. B., Aslan, G., & Aka, P. (2020). An investigation of the effect of the psychoeducation program provided to alexithymic and violent adolescents on the level of alexithymia. *Journal of Child and Adolescent Psychiatric Nursing, 33*(3), 169–179. https://doi.org/10.1111/jcap.12285

Bendig, L. A. W. (1956). The development of a short form of the Manifest anxiety scale. *Journal of Consulting Psychology, 20,* 384. https://doi.org/10.1037/ h0045580

Berenbaum, H., Davis, R., & McGrew, J. (1998). Alexithymia and interpretation of hostile-provoking situations. *Psychotherapy and Psychosomatics, 67,* 254–258. https://doi.org/10.1159/000012288

Berger, J. M., Levant, R. F., McMillan, K. K., Kelleher, W., & Sellers, A. (2005). Impact of gender role conflict, traditional masculinity ideology, alexithymia, and age on men's attitudes toward psychological help seeking. *Psychology of Men and Masculinity, 6,* 73–78. https://doi.org/10.1037/1524-9220.6.1.73

Berke, D. S., Reidy, D., & Zeichner, A. (2018). Masculinity, emotion regulation, and psychopathology: A critical review and integrated model. *Clinical Psychology Review, 66,* 106–116. https://doi.org/10.1016/j.cpr.2018.01.004

Bernstein, E. M., & Putnam, F. W. (1986). Development, reliability, and validity of a dissociative scale. *Journal of Nervous and Mental Disease, 174,* 727–735. https://doi.org/10.1097/00005053-198612000-00004

Blanchard, E. B., Arena, J. G., & Pallmeyer, T. P. (1981). Psychometric properties of a scale to measure alexithymia. *Psychotherapy and Psychosomatics*, *35*, 64–71. https://doi.org/10.1159/000287479

Bosson, J. K., & Vandello, J. A. (2011). Precarious manhood and its links to action and aggression. *Current Directions in Psychological Science, 20*, 82–86. https://doi.org/10.1177/0963721411402669

Brannon, R. (1976). The male sex role: Our culture's blueprint for manhood, what it's done for us lately. In D. David & R. Brannon (Eds.), *The forty-nine percent majority: The male sex role*. Reading, MA: Addison-Wesley.

Bray, L. H. (2003). *Traditional masculinity ideology and normative male alexithymia* (Unpublished doctoral dissertation). University of Alberta.

Bressi, C., Taylor, G., Parker, J., Bressi, S., Brambilla, V., Aguglia, E., et al. (1996). Cross-validation of the 20-item Toronto Alexithymia Scale: An Italian multicenter study. *Journal of Psychosomatic Research*, *41,* 551–559. https://doi.org/10.1016/S0022-3999(96)00228-0

Carpenter, K. M., & Addis, M. E. (2000). Alexithymia, gender, and responses to depressive symptoms. *Sex Roles*, *43,* 629–644. https://doi.org/10.1023/A:1007100523844

Cohen, K., Auld, F., & Brooker, H. (1994). Is alexithymia related to psychosomatic disorder and somaticizing? *Journal of Psychosomatic Research*, *38,* 119–127. https://doi.org/10.1016/0022-3999(94)90085-X

Cohen, R., & Vedantam, S. (2018, March 19). Guys, we have a problem: How American masculinity creates lonely men. *The Hidden Brain*. Retrieved from https://www.npr.org/2018/03/19/594719471/guys-we-have-a-problem-howAmerican-masculinity-creates-lonely-men

Coleman, D., Feigelman, W., & Rosen, Z. (2020). Association of high traditional masculinity and risk of suicide death: Secondary analysis of the Add Health study. *JAMA Psychiatry*, *77*(4), 435–437. https://doi.org/10.1001/jamapsychiatry.2019.4702

Crowne, D. P., & Marlowe, D. (1960). A new scale of social desirability independent of psychopathology. *Journal of Consulting Psychology, 24,* 349–354. https://doi.org/10.1037/h0047358

Dion, K. L. (1996). Ethnolinguistic correlates of alexithymia: Toward a cultural perspective. *Journal of Psychosomatic Research*, *41,* 531–539. https://doi.org/10.1016/S0022-3999(96)00295-4

Eaton, N. R., Keyes, K. M., Krueger, R. F., Balsis, S., Skodol, A. E., Markon, K. E., Grant, B. F., & Hasin, D. S. (2012). An invariant dimensional liability model of gender differences in mental disorder prevalence: Evidence from a national sample. *Journal of Abnormal Psychology, 121*(1), 282–288. https://doi.org/10.1037/a0024780

Forkus, S. R., & Weiss, N. H. (2021). Examining the relations among moral foundations, potentially morally injurious events, and posttraumatic stress disorder symptoms. *Psychological Trauma: Theory, Research, Practice, and Policy, 13*(4), 403–411. https://doi.org/10.1037/tra0000968

Furnham, A., Petrides, K. V., Sisterson, G., & Baluch, B. (2003). Repressive coping style and positive self-presentation. *British Journal of Health Psychology, 8,* 223–249. https://doi.org/10.1348/135910703321649187

Gebhard, K. T., Cattaneo, L. B., Tangney, J. P., Hargrove, S., & Shor, R. (2019). Threatened masculinity shame-related responses among straight men: Measurement and relationship to aggression. *Psychology of Men & Masculinities, 20*(3), 429–444. https://doi.org/10.1037/men0000177

Gerdes, Z. T., Alto, K. M., Jadaszewski, S., D'Auria, F., & Levant, R. F. (2017). A content analysis of research on masculinity ideologies using all forms of the Male Role Norms Inventory (MRNI). *Psychology of Men & Masculinity, 19,* 584–599. https://doi.org/10.1037/men0000134

Gerdes, Z. T., & Levant, R. (2018). Complex relationships among masculine norms and health/well-being outcomes: Correlation patterns of the conformity to masculine normsinventory subscales. *American Journal of Men's Health, 12,* 229–240. https://doi.org/10.1177/1557988317745910

Gough, B., & Robertson, S. (2017). A review of research on men's physical health. In R. F. Levant & Y. J. Wong (Eds.), *The psychology of men and masculinities* (pp. 197–227). Washington, DC: American Psychological Association.

Good, G. E., Wallace, D. L., & Borst, T. S. (1994). Masculinity research: A review and critique. *Applied and Preventive Psychology, 3,* 3–14. https://doi.org/10.1016/S0962-1849(05)80104-0

Haviland, M. G., Hendryx, M. S., Shaw, D. G., & Henry, J. P. (1994). Alexithymia in women and men hospitalized for psychoactive substance dependence. *Comprehensive Psychiatry, 35,* 124–128. https://doi.org/10.1016/0010-440X(94)90056-N

Hedegaard, H., Curtin, S. C., & Warner, M. (2021). Suicide mortality in the United States, 1999-2019. *NCHS Data Brief, 398,* 1–8.

Hendrikx, L. J., & Murphy, D. (2023). Associations between international trauma questionnaire complex posttraumatic stress disorder symptom clusters and moral injury in a sample of UK treatment-seeking veterans: A network approach. *Psychological Trauma: Theory, Research, Practice, and Policy.* https://doi.org/10.1037/tra0001426

Honkalampi, K., Hintakka, J., Tanskanen, A., Lehtonen, J., & Viinamaki, H. (2000). Depression is strongly associated with alexithymia in the general population. *Journal of Psychosomatic Research, 48,* 98–104. https://doi.org/10.1016/S0022-3999(99)00083-5

Hyde, J. S. (2005). The gender similarities hypothesis. *American Psychologist, 60*(6), 581–592. https://doi.org/10.1037/0003-066X.60.6.581

Jardin, E., Allen, P. A., Levant, R. F., Lien, M-C, McCurdy, E. R., Villalba, A., Mallik, P., Houston, J. R., & Gerdes, Z. T. (2019). Event related brain potentials reveal differences in emotional processing in alexithymia. *Journal of Cognitive Psychology, 31,* 619–633. https://doi.org/10.1080/20445911.2019.1642898

Johnson, J. L., Oliffe, J. L., Kelly, M. T., Galdas, P., & Ogrodniczuk, J. S. (2012). Men's discourses of help-seeking in the context of depression. *Sociology of*

Health & Illness, 34(3), 345–361. https://doi.org/10.1111/j.1467-9566.2011 .01372.x

Joseph, S., Williams, R., Irwing, P., & Cammock, T. (1994). The preliminary development of a measure to assess attitudes towards emotional expression. *Personality and Individual Differences, 16,* 869–875. https://doi.org/10.1016 /0191-8869(94)90231-3

Joukamaa, M., Kokkonen, P., Veijola, J., Laksy, K., Karvonen, J. T., Jokelainen, J., et al. (2003). Social situation of expectant mothers and alexithymia 31 years later in their offspring: A prospective study. *Psychosomatic Medicine, 65,* 307–312. https://doi.org/10.1097/01.PSY.0000030389.53353.BC

Joukamaa, M., Sohlman, B., & Lehtinen, V. (1995). The prescription of psychotropic drugs in primary health care. *Acta Psychiatrica Scandinavica, 92,* 359–364. https://doi.org/10.1111/j.1600-0447.1995.tb09597.x

Karakis, E. N., & Levant, R, F. (2012). Is normative male alexithymia associated with relationship satisfaction, fear of intimacy and communication quality among men in heterosexual relationships. *Journal of Men's Studies, 20,* 179–186. https://doi .org/10.3149/jms.2003.179

Kirmayer, L. J., & Robbins, J. M. (1993). Cognitive and social correlates of the Toronto Alexithymia Scale. *Psychosomatics, 34,* 41–52. https://doi.org/10.1016 /S0033-3182(93)71926-X

Kiselica, M. S., & O'Brien, S. (2001, August). Are attachment disorders and alexithymia characteristic of males? In M. S. Kiselica (Chair.), *Are males really emotional mummies? What do the data indicate?* Symposium conducted at the Annual Convention of the American Psychological Association, San Francisco, CA.

Kokkonen, P., Veijola, J., Karvonen, J. T., Laksy, K. Jokelainen, J., Jarvelin, M., et al. (2003). Ability to speak at the age of 1 year and alexithymia 30 years later. *Journal of Psychosonatic Research, 54,* 494–495. https://doi.org/10.1016/ S0022-3999(02)00465-8

Laghai, A., & Joseph, S. (2000). Attitudes towards emotional expression: Factor structure, convergent validity and associations with personality. *British Journal of Medical Psychology, 73,* 381–384. https://doi.org/10.1348/000711200160598

Lane, R. D., Sechrest, L., & Riedel, R. (1998). Sociodemographic correlates of alexithymia. *Comprehensive Psychiatry, 39,* 377–385. https://doi.org/10.1016/ S0010-440X(98)90051-7

Lane, R. D., Sechrest, L., Reidel, R., Weldon, V., Kaszniak, A., & Schwartz, G. E. (1996). Impaired verbal and nonverbal emotion recognition in alexithymia. *Psychosomatic Medicine, 58,* 203–210. https://doi.org/10.1097/00006842 -199605000-00002

Levant, R. F. (1990). Coping with the new father role. In D. Moore & F. Leafgren (Eds.), *Problem solving strategies and interventions for men in conflict* (pp. 81–94). Alexandria, VA: American Association for Counseling and Development.

Levant, R. F. (2011). Research in the psychology of men and masculinity using the gender role strain paradigm as a framework. *American Psychologist, 66,* 765–776. https://doi.org/10.1037/a0025034

Levant, R. F., Allen, P. A., & Lien, M.-C. (2014). Alexithymia in men: How and when does the deficit in the processing of emotions occur? *Psychology of Men and Masculinity, 15,* 324–334. https://doi.org/10.1037/a0033860

Levant, R. F., Good, G. E., Cook, S., O'Neil, J., Smalley, K. B., Owen, K. A., & Richmond, K. (2006). Validation of the normative male Alexithymia scale: Measurement of a gender-linked syndrome. *Psychology of Men and Masculinity, 7,* 212–224. https://doi.org/10.1037/1524-9220.7.4.212

Levant, R. F., Hall, R. J., Williams, C., & Hasan, N. T. (2009). Gender differences in alexithymia: A meta-analysis. *Psychology of Men and Masculinity, 10,* 190–203. https://doi.org/10.1037/a0015652

Levant, R. F., Hirsch, L., Celentano, E., Cozza, T. Hill, S., MacEachern, M., Marty, N., & Schnedeker, J. (1992). The male role: An investigation of contemporary norms. *Journal of Mental Health Counseling, 14,* 325–337.

Levant, R. F., & Kopecky, G. (1995). *Masculinity reconstructed.* New York: Plume.

Levant, R. F., McCurdy, E. R., Keum, B. T. H., Cox, D. W., Halter, M. J., & Stefanov, D. G. (2022, April 7). Mediation and moderation of the relationship between men's endorsement of traditional masculinity ideology and intentions to seek psychotherapy. *Professional Psychology: Research and Practice, 53*(3), 234–243. http://dx.doi.org/10.1037/pro0000461

Levant, R. F., & Richmond, K. (2007). A review of research on masculinity ideologies using the male role norms inventory. *Journal of Men's Studies, 15,* 130–146. *https://doi.org/10.3149/jms.1502.130*

Levant, R. F., & Richmond, K. (2016). The gender role strain paradigm and masculinity ideologies. In Y. J. Wong & S. R. Wester (Eds.), *APA handbook on men and masculinities* (pp. 23–49). Washington, DC: American Psychological Association.

Levant, R. F., Richmond, K., Majors, R. G., Inclan, J. E., Rossello, J. M., Heesacker, et al. (2003). A multicultural investigation of masculinity ideology and alexithymia. *Psychology of Men and Masculinity, 4,* 91–99. https://doi.org/10.1037/1524-9220.4.2.91

Levant, R. F., Rogers, B. K., Cruickshank, B., Kurtz, B. A., Rankin, T. J., Williams, C. M., & Colbow, A, (2012). Exploratory factor analysis and construct validity of the Male Role Norms Inventory-Adolescent-revised (MRNI-A-r). *Psychology of Men and Masculinity, 13,* 354–366. https://doi.org/10.1037/a0029102

Levant, R. F., Webster, B. M., Stanley, J. T., & Thompson, E. (2020). The Aging Men's Masculinity Ideologies Inventory (AMMII): Dimensionality, variance composition, measurement invariance by gender, and validity. *Psychology of Men and Masculinities, 21,* 46–57. http://dx.doi.org/10.1037/men0000208

Levant, R. F., & Wong, Y. J. (2013). Race and gender as moderators of the relationship between the endorsement of traditional masculinity ideology and alexithymia: an intersectional perspective. *Psychology of Men and Masculinity, 14,* 329–333. https://doi.org/10.1037/a0029551

Levant, R. F., Wong, Y. J., Karakis, E. N., & Welch, M. W. (2015). Moderated mediation of the relationship between the endorsement of restrictive emotionality and alexithymia. *Psychology of Men and Masculinity, 16,* 459–467. https://doi.org/10.3758/s13428-013-0434-y

Litz, B. T., Stein, N., Delaney, E., Lebowitz, L., Nash, W. P., Silva, C., & Maguen, S. (2009). Moral injury and moral repair in war veterans: A preliminary model and intervention strategy. *Clinical Psychology Review*, *29*(8), 695–706. https://doi.org /10.1016/j.cpr.2009.07.003

Loas, G., Corcos, M., Stephan, P., Pellet, J., Bizouard, P., & Venisse, J. L. (2001). Factorial structure of the 20-item Toronto Alexithymia Scale confirmatory factorial analysis in nonclinical and clinical samples. *Journal of Psychosomatic Research*, *50*, 255–261. https://doi.org/10.1016/S0022-3999(01)00197-0

Lumley, M. A., & Sielky, K. (2000). Alexithymia, gender, and hemispheric functioning. *Comprehensive Psychiatry*, *41*, 352–359. https://doi.org/10.1053/comp.2000 .9014

MacArthur, H. J., & Shields, S. A. (2015). There's no crying in baseball, or is there? Male athletes, tears, and masculinity in North America. *Emotion Review*, *7*(1), 39–46. https://doi.org/10.1177/1754073914544476

Mahalik, J. R., & Di Bianca, M. (2021). Help-seeking for depression as a stigmatized threat to masculinity. *Professional Psychology: Research and Practice*, *52*(2), 146–155. https://doi.org/10.1037/pro0000365

Mahalik, J. R., Good, G. E., & Englar-Carlson, M. (2003). Masculinity scripts, presenting concerns and help-seeking: Implications for practice and training. *Professional Psychology: Theory, Research and Practice*, *34*, 123–131. https:// doi.org/10.1037/0735-7028.34.2.123

Mahalik, J. R., Lagan, H. D., & Morrison, J. A. (2006). Health behaviors and masculinity in Kenyan and U.S. male college students. *Psychology of Men & Masculinity, 7*(4), 191–202.

Mattila, A. K., Keefer, K. V., Taylor, G. J., Joukamaa, M., Jula, A., Parker, J. D. A., & Bagby, R. M. (2010). Taxometric analysis of alexithymia in a general population sample from Finland. *Personality and Individual Differences*, *49*, 216–221. https:// doi.org/10.1016/j.paid.2010.03.038

McCallum, M., Piper, W. E., Ogrodniczuk, J. S., & Joyce, A. S. (2003). Relationships among psychological mindedness, alexithymia, and outcome in four forms of short-term psychotherapy. *Psychology and Psychotherapy: Theory, Research and Practice, 76*, 133–144. https://doi.org/10.1348/147608303765951177

McDermott, R. C., Smith, P. N., Borgogna, N., Booth, N., Granato, S., & Sevig, T. D. (2018). College students' conformity to masculine role norms and help-seeking intentions for suicidal thoughts. *Psychology of Men & Masculinity*, *19*(3), 340–351. https://doi.org/10.1037/men0000107

Mendolia, M. (2002). An index of self-regulation of emotion and the study of repression in social contexts that threaten or do not threaten self-concept. *Emotion*, *2*, 215–232. https://doi.org/10.1037/1528-3542.2.3.215

Millard, R. W., & Kinsler, B. J. (1992). Evaluation of constricted affect in chronic pain: An attempt using the Toronto Alexythymia (SIC) Scale. *Pain, 50*, 287–292. https://doi.org/10.1016/0304-3959(92)90033-8

Myers, L. B., & Derakshan, N. (2004). The repressive coping style and avoidance of negative affect. In I. Nyklicek, L. Temoshok, & A. Vingerhoets (Eds.), *Emotional expression and health: Advances in theory, assessment and clinical applications* (pp. 169–184). New York: Brunner-Routledge.

Ogrodniczuk, J. S., Piper, W. E., & Joyce, A. S. (2004). Alexithymia as a predictor of residual symptoms in depressed patients who respond to short-term psychotherapy. *American Journal of Psychotherapy*, *82*, 469–473.

O'Neil, J. M. (1981). Male sex role conflicts, sexism, and masculinity: Psychological implications for men, women, and the counseling psychologist. *The Counseling Psychologist, 9*(2), 61–79. https://doi.org/10.1177/001100008100900213

O'Neil, J. M. (2008). Summarizing 25 years of research on men's gender role conflict using the gender role conflict scale. *The Counseling Psychologist, 36,* 358–445. https://doi.org/10.1177/0011000008317057

O'Neil, J. M., Helms, B., Gable, R. David, L., & Wrightsman, L. (1986). Gender-role conflict scale: College men's fear of femininity. *Sex Roles*, *14*(5/6), 335–350. https://doi.org/10.1007/BF00287583

O'Neil, J. M., Wester, S., Vogel, D., & Danforth, L. (2012). Development and evaluation of the Gender Role Conflict Scale Short Form (GRCS-SF). *Psychology of Men and Masculinity*, *13*, 199–210. https://doi.org/10.1037/a0025550

Pandey, R., Mandal, M. K., Taylor, G. J., & Parker, J. D. A. (1996). Cross-cultural alexithymia: Development and validation of a Hindi translation of the 20-item Toronto Alexithymia Scale. *Journal of Clinical Psychology, 52,* 173–176. https://doi.org/10.1002/(SICI)1097-4679(199603)52:2<173::AID-JCLP8>3.0.CO;2-V

Parker, J. A., Bagby, R. M., Taylor, G. J., Endler, N. S., & Schmitz, P. (1993). Factorial validity of the 20-item Toronto Alexithymia Scale. *European Journal of Personality*, *7*, 221–232. Retrieved from ebscohost.com. https://doi.org/10.1002/per.2410070403

Parker, J. D. A., Keefer, K. V., Taylor, G. J., & Bagby, R. M. (2008). Latent structure of the alexithymia construct: A taxometric investigation. *Psychological Assessment*, *20*, 385–396. https://doi.org/10.1037/a0014262

Parker, J. D. A., Taylor, G. J., & Bagby, R. M. (1989). The alexithymia construct: Relationship with sociodemographic variables and intelligence. *Comprehensive Psychiatry, 30,* 434–441. https://doi.org/10.1016/0010-440X(89)90009-6

Parker, J. D. A., Taylor, G. J., & Bagby, R. M. (2001). The relationship between emotional intelligence and alexithymia. *Personality and Individual Differences*, *30*, 107–115. https://doi.org/10.1016/S0191-8869(00)00014-3

Parker, J. D. A., Taylor, G. J., & Bagby, R. M. (1993a). Alexithymia and the recognition of facial expressions of emotion. *Psychotherapy and Psychosomatics, 59,* 197–202. https://doi.org/10.1159/000288664

Parker, J. D. A., Taylor, G. J., & Bagby, R. M. (1993b). Alexithymia and the processing of emotional stimuli: An experimental study. *New Trends in Experimental and Clinical Psychiatry, 9,* 9–14.

Parker, J. A., Taylor, G. J., & Bagby, R. M. (2003). The 20-item Toronto Alexithymia Scale III. Reliability and factorial validity in a community population. *Journal of Psychosomatic Research, 55,* 269–275. https://doi.org/10.1016/S0022-3999(02)00578-0

Pasini, A., Delle Chiaie, D., Seripa, S., & Ciani, N. (1992). Alexithymia as related to sex, age, and educational level: Results of the Toronto Alexithymia Scale in 417 normal subjects. *Comprehensive Psychiatry*, *33,* 42–46. https://doi.org/10.1016 /0010-440X(92)90078-5

Plan International USA. (2018). *The state of gender equality for U.S. Adolescents.* Retrieved from https://www.planusa.org/docs/state-of-gender-equality -summary-2018.pdf

Pleck, J. H. (1981). *The myth of masculinity.* Cambridge, MA: MIT Press.

Pleck, J. H. (1995). The gender role strain paradigm: An update. In R. F. Levant & W. S. Pollack (Eds.), *A new psychology of men* (pp. 11–32). New York: Basic Books.

Pollack, W. S. (1998). *Real boys: Rescuing our sons from the myths of boyhood.* New York: Random House.

Porcelli, P., & Taylor, G. J. (2018). Alexithymia and physical illness: A psychosomatic approach. In O. Luminet, R. M. Bagby, & G. J. Taylor (Eds.), *Alexithymia: Advances in research, theory, and clinical practice* (pp. 105–126). Cambridge University Press. https://doi.org/10.1017/9781108241595.009

Prince, J. D., & Berenbaum, H. (1993). Alexithymia and hedonic capacity. *Journal of Research in Personality*, *27*, 15–22. https://doi.org/10.1006/jrpe.1993.1002

Pryor, S. M. (2023). *The problem and the solution: Exploring factors related to masculinity and self-stigma associated with seeking psychological help* (Unpublished doctoral dissertation). The University of Akron.

Radloff, L. S. (1977). The CES-D scale: A self-report depression scale for research in the general population. *Applied Psychological Measurement*, *1*, 385–401. https:// doi.org/10.1177/014662167700100306

Ramaeker, J., & Petrie, T. A. (2019). "Man up!": Exploring intersections of sport participation, masculinity, psychological distress, and help-seeking attitudes and intentions. *Psychology of Men & Masculinities, 20*(4), 515–527. https://doi.org/10 .1037/men0000198

Saarijärvi, S., Salminen, J. K., Tamminen, T., & Äärelä, E. (1993). Alexithymia in psychiatric consultation-liason patients. *General Hospital Psychiatry*, *15*, 330–333. https://doi.org/10.1016/0163-8343(93)90026-K

Salminen, J. K., Saarijarvi, S., Aarela, E., Toikka, T., & Kauhanen, J. (1999). *Journal of Psychosomatic Research, 46,* 75–82. https://doi.org/10.1016/S0022 -3999(98)00053-1

Shields, S. A. (2013). Gender and emotion: What we think we know, what we need to know, and why it matters. *Psychology of Women Quarterly*, *37*(4), 423–435. https://doi.org/10.1177/0361684313502312

Suslow, T., & Junghanns, K. (2002). Impairments of emotion situation priming in alexithymia. *Personality and Individual Differences*, *32,* 541–550. https://doi.org /10.1016/S0191-8869(01)00056-3

Taylor, G. H., Bagby, R. M., Ryan, D. P., Parker, J. D. A., Doody, F. F., & Keefe, P. (1988). Criterion validity of the Toronto Alexithymia Scale. *Psychosomatic Medicine*, *50*, 500–509. https://doi.org/10.1097/00006842-198809000-00006

Taylor, G. J. (2004). Alexithymia: Twenty-five years of theory and research. In I. Nyklicek, L. Temoshok, & A. Vingerhoets. (Eds.), *Emotional expression and* health: Advances in theory, assessment and clinical applications (pp. 137–153). New York: Brunner-Routledge.

Taylor, J. A. (1953). A personality scale of manifest anxiety. Journal of Abnormal and Social Psychology, 48, 285–290. https://doi.org/10.1037/h0056264

Taylor, G. J., Parker, J. D. A., Bagby, R. M., & Acklin, M. W. (1992). Alexithymia and somatic complaints in psychiatric outpatients. Journal of Psychosomatic Research, 46, 417–424. https://doi.org/10.1016/0022-3999(92)90002-J

Taylor, G. J., Parker, J. D. A., Bagby, R. M., & Bourke, M. P. (1996). Relationships between alexithymia and psychological characteristics associated with eating disorder. Journal of Psychosomatic Research, 41, 561–568. https://doi.org/10.1016/S0022-3999(96)00224-3

Taylor, G. J., Ryan, D., & Bagby, R. M. (1985). Toward the development of a new self-report alexithymia scale. Psychotherapy and Psychosomatics, 44, 191–199. https://doi.org/10.1159/000287912

Terlizzi, E. P., & Zablotsky, B. (2020). Mental health treatment among adults: United States, 2019 (NCHS Data Brief, No 380). National Center for Health Statistics.

Todarello, O., Taylor, G. J., Parker, J. D. A., & Fanelli, M. (1995). Alexithymia in essential hypertensive and psychiatric outpatients: A comparative study. Journal of Psychosomatic Research, 39, 987–994. https://doi.org/10.1016/0022-3999(95)00506-4

Van Ijzendoorn, M. H., & Schuengel, C. (1996). The measurement of dissociation in normal and clinical populations: Meta-analytic validation of the dissociative experiences scale (DES). Clinical Psychology Review, 16(5), 365–382. https://doi.org/10.1016/0272-7358(96)00006-2

Vingerhoets, A. J. J. M., Van Heck, G. L., Grim, R., & Bermond, B. (1995). Alexithymia: A further exploration of its nomological network. Psychotherapy and Psychosomatics, 64, 32–42. https://doi.org/10.1159/000288988

Watson, D., & Clark, L. A. (1994). The PANAS-X: Manual for the positive and negative affect schedule - expanded form. Iowa City: The University of Iowa Press.

Weigard, A., Loviska, A. M., & Beltz, A. M. (2021). Little evidence for sex or ovarian hormone influences on affective variability. Scientific Reports, 11(1), 1–12. https://doi.org/10.1038/s41598-021-00143-7

Wester, S. R., Vogel, D. L., Pressly, P. K., & Heesacker, M. (2002). Sex differences in emotion: A critical review of the literature and implications for counseling psychology. The Counseling Psychologist, 30(4), 630–652. https://doi.org/10.1177/00100002030004008

Wise, T. N., Mann, L. S., & Shay, L. (1992). Alexithymia and the five-factor model of personality. Comprehensive Psychiatry, 3, 147–151. https://doi.org/10.1016/0010-440X(92)90023-J

Wong, Y. J., Ho, M.-H. R., Wang, S.-Y., & Miller, I. S. K. (2017). Meta-analyses of the relationship between conformity to masculine norms and mental health-related outcomes. Journal of Counseling Psychology, 64(1), 80–93. https://doi.org/10.1037/cou0000176

Wong, Y. J., Pituch, K. A., & Rochlen, A. B. (2006). Men's restrictive emotionality: An investigation of associations with other emotion-related constructs, anxiety and underlying dimensions. *Psychology of Men and Masculinity*, *7*, 113–126. https://doi.org/10.1037/1524-9220.7.2.113

Yelsma, P., Hovestadt, A. J., Anderson, W. T., & Nilsson, J. W. (2000). Family of origin expressiveness: Measurement, meaning, and relationship to alexithymia. *Journal of Marital and Family Therapy*, *3*, 353–363. https://doi.org/10.1111/j.1752-0606.2000.tb00304.x

Zeitlin, S. B., & McNally, R. J. (1993). Alexithymia and anxiety sensitivity in panic disorder and obsessive-compulsive disorder. *American Journal of Psychiatry*, *150*, 658–660. https://doi.org/10.1176/ajp.150.4.658

Zenger, J., & Folkman, J. (2019, June 25). Research: Women score higher than men in most leadership skills. *Harvard Business Review*. Retrieved from https://hbr.org/2019/06/research-women-score-higher-than-men-in-most-leadership-skills

PART II

Assessment

If you are a clinician reading this book, you may have a client or two in mind whom you suspect might benefit from ART. However, it can be difficult to ascertain whether they might be alexithymic and to what degree. The chapters in Part II seek to present scales that can be used in the office to assess for alexithymia.

For those who may be unfamiliar with scale development, it is important to understand the basics on how scales are built and refined over time. In the coming chapters, specific details on each scale's development and refinement will be provided; however, if you are uninterested or unfamiliar with this process, such information might appear overwhelming. To make it feel less so, here is a simplified description of the process: scales start out as a large list of potential statements that capture the essence of what the researcher is interested in measuring. These statements can be compiled by interviewing members of the target group, or by reviewing prior literature, or both. That list then undergoes a rigorous vetting process, and a final list of preliminary items are tested on a sample of interest. The tested items are then subjected to various statistical analyses to determine if they measure what they are supposed to be measuring (i.e., is the scale valid?) and if they are consistent (i.e., is the scale reliable). If all goes well, then the scale is published. Following publication, that scale is continuously tested throughout the years and compared to other similar scales to determine if it remains usable in the present day. If it is not, it is either revised or replaced by an entirely new scale.

It is common for scales to undergo revision over the years. We will see that in future chapters with the Normative Male Alexithymia Scale (NMAS; Levant et al., 2006), and the Normative Male Alexithymia Scale- Brief Form (NMAS-BF). Using updated statistical techniques, the NMAS-BF, which was significantly reduced from its parent scale of 29-items to only 6-items, was found to be just as effective, if not more, at assessing Normative Male Alexithymia in a fraction of the time. This allows clinicians to assess for alexithymia quickly and accurately.

Regardless of your level of competence regarding scale development, it is important to know that the scientific process is critical in forging instruments that reliably and validly measure what they are intended to measure, in this case, alexithymia. Clinicians should only use scientifically supported instruments in their work with clients to allow for accurate assessment and treatment planning. The information provided in the coming chapters discusses the scale development process in three effective measures of alexithymia, the Toronto Alexithymia Scale-20 (TAS-20; Bagby et al., 1994), the NMAS, and the NMAS-BF. The NMAS is provided at the end of its chapter for the reader's use, and the NMAS-BF is included in both Alexithymia Reduction Treatment manuals. To get the TAS-20, write to the scale developer Graeme J. Taylor: graeme.taylor@utoronto.ca

Variance Composition, Reliability, Validity, and Measurement Invariance of the Toronto Alexithymia Scale-20 in Non-clinical Samples[1]

Ronald F. Levant, Mike C. Parent, Shu Ling, and Nicholas C. Borgogna

INTRODUCTION

The purpose of the present study was to assess the evidence for using the total scale score of the Toronto Alexithymia Scale-20 (TAS-20; Bagby et al., 1994). This is an important task, because recent research has pointed to the "hidden invalidity" of many psychological scales, with particular reference to structural validity – i.e., dimensionality (factor structure) and measurement equivalence/ invariance (Hussey & Hughes, 2020). The TAS-20 total raw scale score is often used in research in the psychology of men and masculinities (PMM), as well as in clinical practice, largely because of prior research establishing criteria for its use in diagnosing alexithymia (Taylor et al., 1988), until recently the only such scale to have done so. However, the Bermond-Vorst Alexithymia Questionnaire-20 was recently subjected to such an analysis "based on the sensitivity, specificity, receiver operating characteristic curve analysis, and the analyses of the clinical data" (Loas et al., 2015, p. 1). In examining how Alexithymia is diagnosed, newer scales have been developed over the last ten years which move away from classifying someone as either "alexithymia" or "non-alexithymic." Preece and colleagues (2018) created the Perth Alexithymia Questionnaire (PAQ), which demonstrated capabilities to measure whether one scored in the low, average, or high range in alexithymia, making the construct more of a spectrum.

DOI: 10.4324/9781003378518-6

Empirical support for the use of the total raw scale score would require a demonstration that, despite the intended multi-dimensional nature of the scale, it can be used as unidimensional measure of alexithymia. This demonstration might involve confirmatory factor analytic (CFA) results confirming the existence of either a unidimensional structure, in which the items load only on a general alexithymia factor, or a bifactor structure, in which the items load on both their group factors (corresponding to the subscales) and a general alexithymia factor (corresponding to the total scale score), or a hierarchical structure, in which the items load only on their first order factor (corresponding to the subscale scores), which in turn load on the second order factor (corresponding to the total scale score). To conduct this investigation, the variance composition of the TAS-20 was examined, and model-based reliability and omega coefficients were calculated. In addition, evidence for the validity of a unidimensional TAS-20 for men was assessed. Finally, measurement invariance of the unidimensional TAS-20 by gender was assessed.

Prior Examination of the Psychometric Properties of the TAS-20

The TAS-20 is the most popular scale for alexithymia assessment (Gignac et al., 2007; Meganck et al., 2008; Preece et al., 2017; Reise et al., 2013a). It has been used extensively worldwide. One reason for the scale's popularity is that the scale developers established criteria based on clinical research for determining the presence or absence of alexithymia using TAS-20 scores (Taylor et al., 1988), in which scores > 61 indicated the presence of alexithymia, and scores < 51 indicated the absence of alexithymia. Given this advantage other scales were used much less frequently.

However, significant psychometric problems with the scale have been reported. The first confirmatory factor analysis (CFA) reported a three-factor common (or correlated) factors model (in which items load only on the factors corresponding to the subscales), with the factors corresponding to the three theorized dimensions – difficulty identifying feelings (DIF), difficulty describing feelings (DDF), and externally oriented thinking (EOT) (Parker et al., 1993). However, Parker et al. (1993) used fit statistics that have been criticized for their dependence on sample size (Hu & Bentler, 1998), and with values that do not meet contemporary criteria (i.e., GFI = .886, AGFI = .856). A decade later, Parker et al. (2003) reported a CFA using the common factors model with a mixed gender sample, finding adequate fit (GFI = .98, AGFI = .98, CFI = .97, RMSEA = .06). However, these results do not support the use of the total scale score and conflict with those of a series of other studies.

Several psychometric studies found that the first two factors (DIF, DDF) collapsed into one (Erni et al., 1997; Kooimana et al., 2002; Loas et al.,1996).

Furthermore, evidence for the dimensionality and reliability of the EOT scale has also been questioned (Gignac et al., 2007; Meganck et al., 2008; Preece et al., 2017). In a review, Kooimana et al. (2002, p. 1083) noted that "in practically all studies the dimension 'externally oriented thinking' (EOT) appears to be unreliable." As a result, several different approaches have been taken with regard to EOT, including breaking EOT into two subscales (Haviland & Reise, 1996; Meganck et al., 2008; Ritz & Kannapin, 2000), and also creating a method factor to account for the fact that all but one of the negatively-keyed items load on the EOT factor (Gignac et al., 2007; Meganck et al., 2008). Thus, the dimensional structure of the TAS-20 is questionable.

Four studies assessed the dimensional structure of the TAS-20. First, Gignac et al. (2007) tested common factors and hierarchical models specifying the original three subscales, and four bifactor models. The latter had a general alexithymia factor plus one of several sets of group factors. Of all the models tested, only one model had acceptable levels of incremental fit and good levels of absolute fit; however the required covariance link can only be accomplished using structural equation modeling (SEM), precluding the use of raw scores. Second, Meganck et al. (2008), using both clinical and student samples, found unacceptable fit for a unidimensional model. Two of three hierarchical models tested had worse fit than their respective common factors models. These models specified a second order factor and one of two sets of first order factors: 1. original three subscales; 2. combining DIF and DDF and splitting EOT into two factors. A third hierarchical model with separate DIF and DDF factors and splitting EOT into two factors had equivocal fit. Third, Preece et al. (2017) tested one unidimensional model, four common factors models, and three hierarchical models. They found that the hierarchical models resulted in decrements in fit as compared to their common factors counterparts in both samples, and all had unacceptable fit statistics. Finally, Tuliao et al. (2019) examined 19^2 factor structures in two samples, from the US and the Philippines. Only one model in both samples met the criteria for acceptable fit criteria, and this was the only model that dropped items, suggesting that model trimming may be the way to improve the scale's psychometric properties.

Finally, Reise et al. (2013a) took a very different approach to studying the dimensionality of the TAS-20, deploying new psychometric indices (e.g., model-based dimensionality and reliability indices) to determine the extent that the TAS-20 total scale scores can be reliably reported. They found "compelling evidence that the item responses are 'essentially unidimensional'" (p. 138). As will be discussed, while the present study replicates dimensionality and reliability analyses conducted by Reise et al. (2013a), it goes beyond it in also assessing evidence for validity in men using latent variables and measurement invariance by gender.

THE PRESENT STUDY

The first aim was to assess the dimensionality of the TAS-20 by estimating its fit to the data in unidimensional, common factors, bifactor and hierarchical models. The second aim was to assess the scale's dimensionality and the reliability of the total scale and subscale scores using the technique utilized by Reise et al. (2013a), namely calculating model-based dimensionality and reliability coefficients. Based on Reise et al. (2013a), we hypothesized (**H1**) that this analysis will provide evidence for a unidimensional structure. The third aim was to assess the validity of the TAS-20 in men. Validity information for the TAS-20 based on raw scores is abundant (c.f., Taylor, 2004), but we are not aware of any studies that provide TAS-20 validity evidence for men using latent variables, which is a more stringent method as it removes many sources of error. Thus, this aim was to assess the convergent construct and concurrent criterion-related evidence for the validity of the TAS-20 using a latent variable approach. A CFA model which regressed the TAS-20 model on several related latent constructs was estimated.

To assess convergent construct evidence for validity, the gender-linked Normative Male Alexithymia Scale (NMAS) was used. The NMAS has been moderately associated with the TAS-20 (Levant et al., 2006). Hence, we hypothesized (**H2**) that the TAS-20 will be significantly, moderately, and positively related to the NMAS.

Conceptually, alexithymia should be inversely related to the ability to identify and describe one's emotions toward others and oneself. Two scales were used to assess concurrent criterion-related evidence for validity by these dimensions. To assess the relationship between alexithymia and emotional identification/description toward others, we used the Revised Adult Attachment Scale (RAAS), which has three subscales: Close, Depend, and Anxiety (Collins & Read, 1990). Previous research has found a moderate, negative relationship between alexithymia and relationship satisfaction (Humphreys et al., 2009). Furthermore, the NMAS (closely linked to the TAS-20) has been found to have small negative correlations with relationship consensus, cohesion, satisfaction, and affectional expression, and a moderately positive one with fear of intimacy (Karakis & Levant, 2012). Therefore, based on the above-defined conceptualization of alexithymia and on previous research, we hypothesized that the TAS-20 would have significant, small, and negative correlations with the Close Scale of the RAAS (**H3**), which measures the extent to which a person is comfortable with closeness and intimacy and to the Depend scale of the RAAS (**H4**), which measures the extent to which a person feels they can depend on others to be available when needed. We also hypothesized that the TAS-20 would demonstrate a significant, small, and positive correlation with the Anxiety scale, which measures the extent to which a person is worried about being abandoned (**H5**).

We additionally wanted to extend the convergent evidence for the validity of the TAS-20 by examining how it would be related to a measure of emotional identification/description toward aspects of oneself. To do this, we used the Body Appreciation Scale (BAS; Avalos et al., 2005). Conceptually, individuals higher in alexithymia should demonstrate less emotional identification/description toward themselves, such as in regard to their body image. By extension, the TAS-20 should be inversely correlated with the body appreciation. Prior research supports this position, as Leone et al. (2015) showed that men likely to have alexithymia (as measured by the TAS-20) were also more likely to demonstrate symptoms of muscle dysphoria. Hence, we hypothesized (**H6**) that the TAS-20 would be significantly, small-to-moderately, and negatively correlated with the BAS.

The final aim was to assess the measurement invariance of the TAS-20 across gender (men, women).

METHOD

Participants (Sample 1)

Sample 1 was drawn from a larger project (Levant et al., 2014). A total of 913 university students were included in the analysis (73.4% men and 26.6% women[3]). Participants' age ranged from 18 to 54 years, with a mean of 20.88 (SD = 4.44). Women and men did not differ in mean age. Most participants identified as White (79.4%), however 14.1% identified as Black, 3.6% as Middle Eastern, 3.5% as Asian/Asian American, 2.8% as Latinx, 1.9% as American Indians, 0.2% as Pacific Islanders, and 0.6% as other. Most participants were heterosexual (91.8%), yet 3.6% were gay/lesbian, 3.2% were bisexual, and 1.4% identified either as "other" or did not answer.

Participants (Sample 2)

Sample 2 was drawn from a larger project (Parent & Bradstreet, 2019). A total of 505 men were included in the analysis. Participants age ranged from 19 to 73 years, with a mean of 35.28 (SD = 11.08). Regarding race/ethnicity, most participants identified as White (73.9%), but 11.3% identified as Asian or Asian American, 5.1% as Black, 4.8% as multiracial, 3.2% as Hispanic, 1.6% as either American Indian or did not respond. Most (90.3%) participants identified as heterosexual, but 4.2% indicated they were bisexual, 3.6% indicated they were gay, and 2.0% indicated a different identity or did not respond.

Recruitment and Survey Procedures

For sample 1, the study was approved by the first author's university Institutional Review Board (IRB). University students were recruited using departmental undergraduate research participation pools. Using Qualtrics, after completing the informed consent, participants filled out the questionnaires, and were provided with an educational debriefing. Following completion of the study, participants were redirected to another Qualtrics site where they could confidentially enter their information to receive course credit.

For sample 2, the study was approved by the second author's university IRB. Community-dwelling participants were recruited using Amazon's Mechanical Turk (Mturk) service. Access to the survey was restricted to individuals in the United States who had 95% or better approval on prior Mturk tasks. Using Qualtrics, after completing the informed consent, participants filled out the questionnaires, and were provided with a debriefing. The survey contained two attention checks; those who did not answer the attention check items correctly were exited from the survey and their data were not used. Following completion, a payment of $1.00 was credited to participants' MTurk accounts.

Sample Size Considerations

For the CFAs required for the assessment of variance composition and calculation of model-based reliability and omega coefficients, Kline (2016) recommended a minimum of ten participants for every freely estimated parameter. The bifactor CFA had the largest number of parameters at 80, requiring 800 participants. Our n of 913 exceeded this number. The validity analysis using structural regression had 69 parameters, requiring 690 participants. Our n of 505 was less than this number and may not be adequate. However, using Soper's (2013) *a priori* sample size calculator for structural equation models, with a small effect size of .20, power of .8, six latent variables, 18 observed variables, and $p < .05$, a sample size of 403 is sufficient. Finally, for the analysis of measurement invariance, the largest number of parameters for the basic test had 60 parameters, requiring 600 participants, for which our n of 913 was more than sufficient.

Measures

Toronto Alexithymia Scale-20 (TAS-20)

The TAS-20 (Parker et al., 1993) was created to assess alexithymia. Exploratory factor analysis supported a three-factor structure: DIF, DDF, and EOT, although (as detailed above) subsequent CFAs indicate that the dimensionality is not clear. Participants respond to items using a five-point Likert scale (1 = *strongly disagree*; 5 = *strongly agree*). Internal consistency has been shown to be reliable (Parker et al., 1993). The TAS-20 was found to be positively correlated with measures of somatic complaints (Taylor et al.,1992).

Normative Male Alexithymia Scale (NMAS)

The NMAS (Levant et al., 2006) is a 20-item inventory designed to assess a gender-linked form of alexithymia – Normative Male Alexithymia. Participants answered questions about their own experience of emotions on a seven-point scale (1 = *strongly disagree*; 7 = *strongly agree*). Seven items are reverse-scored. A mean is taken, with higher scores indicating greater Normative Male Alexithymia. EFA and CFA using separate samples indicated that the NMAS consisted of a single 20-item factor. Men's scores on the NMAS displayed very good internal consistency and test-retest reliability over a 1–2 month period. Results of analyses of sex differences, relations of the NMAS with other instruments, and its incremental validity in predicting masculinity ideology provided evidence supporting validity.

Revised Adult Attachment Scale (RAAS)

The RAAS (Collins & Read, 1990) is an 18-item inventory designed to assess adult romantic relationships along three dimensions: Close, Depend, and Anxiety. High scores on the Close scale characterize individuals who are comfortable with closeness and intimacy (Collins, 1996). Participants rated their feelings about romantic relationships using a five-point scale (1 = *not at all characteristic of me*, 5 = *very characteristic of me*). A review of 25 instruments on attachment found that compared with other instruments, RAAS had good test-retest, internal consistency, and inter-item reliability, and good convergent and discriminant validity (Ravitz et al., 2010). The test-retest reliabilities for the three subscales range from .52 to .71 (Collins & Read, 1990). The internal consistency of the subscales have been shown to be > .76 (Eng et al., 2001).

Body Appreciation Scale (BAS)

The BAS (Avalos et al., 2005) is a 13-item measure that examines four related components of positive body image: Holding positive opinions of the body, acceptance of the body despite its imperfections, respect for the body, and protection of the body through the rejection of unrealistic ideals. All items were rated on a five-point scale (1 = *never*; 5 = *always*). Higher scores indicate more positive body image. The internal consistency of the measure has been supported with a non-clinical sample: Cronbach's α = .94 (Avalos et al., 2005). It shows good test-retest reliability (Avalos et al., 2005), and gender equivalence (Tylka, 2013). BAS scores have been shown to be correlated with men's muscularity dissatisfaction, body fat dissatisfaction, height dissatisfaction, and overall body dissatisfaction (Tylka, 2013).

Data Analytic Procedures

We first estimated unidimensional, common factors, bifactor and hierarchical models of the TAS-20. Second, following the recommendations of Reise et al. (2013a), we calculated model-based reliability and omega coefficients to assess the TAS-20's dimensionality, which required entering the standardized factor loadings for both the unidimensional and bifactor models into a model-based reliability calculator developed by Dueber (2017). For the CFAs and the testing of hypotheses 1 through 6, we used M*plus* v.8.3 (Muthén & Muthén, 1998–2015) SEM software. The overall fit of any CFA models was assessed with the scaled chi-square goodness-of-fit test. However, because this statistic is dependent on sample size, it is overly sensitive to trivial sources of model misfit when sample sizes are large (Cheung & Rensvold, 2002). Thus, we used a set of alternative fit indices to determine whether a model demonstrates adequate fit (Kahn, 2006). Acceptable model fit is indicated by the comparative fit (CFI) and Tucker-Lewis fit indices (TLI) over .90, root mean square error of approximation (RMSEA) under .08, and standardized root mean square residual (SRMR) under .10. Good fit is indicated by a CFI and TLI over .95, RMSEA under .05, and SRMR under .05.

For the assessment of measurement invariance, the fits of nested CFA models were compared using a scaled chi-square difference test, which was adjusted for the use of the maximum likelihood estimation with robust standard errors (MLR; Satorra & Bentler, 1999). However, similar to the chi-square goodness-of-fit test, the scaled chi-square difference test ($\Delta\chi2$) is affected by large sample sizes (Cheung & Lau, 2012; Cheung & Rensvold, 2002). Since the $\Delta\chi2$ is expected to be statistically significant in samples larger than 300 (Kline, 2016), we also utilized a ΔCFI with a cut-off score of < .01 (Chen, 2007; Cheung & Lau, 2012; Cheung & Rensvold, 2002).

The descriptive statistics were calculated using SPSS 25. For the validity hypotheses we followed the recommendations of Russell et al. (1998), and created three-to-four-item parcels from the manifest variables for each instrument or subscale that had six or more observed items. Item parcels were created by performing principle axis exploratory factor analyses with one-factor solutions for the items comprising each scale. Iterative assignment of items into one of the parcels was done to ensure that parcel loadings were balanced. Effect sizes were graded according to Ferguson's (2009) criteria for strength of association, where .2 = small, .5 = moderate, and .8 = large.

RESULTS

Before data analyses, both samples were checked for ineligible participants, outliers, normality, and missing data.

Assessment of Dimensionality and Reliability

Dimensionality

As noted above, we first conducted CFA's modeling the TAS-20 as common factors, bifactor, hierarchical and unidimensional models. In the bifactor model all factors were constrained to be orthogonal to each other to allow the uncontaminated assessment of sources of variance in each item. As expected from prior research, none of the models fit well, although the bifactor model had the best fit. See Table 4.1 for fit statistics. Ordinarily, we would follow recommended procedures to trim composite measurement scales (c.f. Goetz et al., 2013) to improve the model fit; however, copyright restrictions prevented us from doing that (Taylor, personal communication, February 1, 2021).

Given that the fit of the bifactor model was adequate in regard to RMSEA and SRMR and only marginally inadequate in regard to CFI (CFI = .89, RMSEA = .065 [.060, .070], and SRMR = .052), the standardized factor loadings for both the unidimensional and bifactor models were then entered into Dueber's (2017) model-based dimensionality and reliability calculator. Table 4.2 summarizes the results. With regard to dimensionality, using the Reise et al. (2013b) criteria, we missed the criterion of high Percentage of Uncontaminated Correlations (PUC) (> .80), which would have meant low risk of parameter bias if it had been met. However, Reise et al. (2013b) also stated that low PUC (< .80; ours was

TABLE 4.1 Model Fit Statistics and Comparisons of Single-Group TAS-20 Models

Single-Group Model	χ^2 (df)	CFI, TLI	RMSEA estimate & 90% CI	SRMR
SG1: Common Factors	531.72 (167)	.697, .655	.098 [.089, .108]	.092
SG2: Bifactor	731.66 (150)	.888, .858	.065 [.060, .070]	.052
SG3: Hierarchical	531.72 (167)	.697, .655	.098 [.089, .108]	.092
SG4: Unidimensional	1499.74 (170)	.744, .714	.093 [.088, .097]	.086
Comparison	$\Delta\chi^2$(df)	p	ΔCFI	Conclusion
SG1 vs. SG2	79.48(17)	.00001	+.19	Prefer SG2

Note. CFI = Comparative Fit Index; TLI = Tucker-Lewis Index; RMSEA = Root Mean Square Error of Approximation; SRMR = Standardized Root Mean Square Residual.

TABLE 4.2 Explained Common Variance and Model-Based Reliability Estimates for the TAS-20

	General	DIF	DDF	EOT
ECV	.66	.19	.20	.80
Omega	.89	.90	.80	.59
Omega H	.76	–	–	–
Omega H S	–	.15	.16	.47
Relative Omega	.86	.16	.20	.79

Note. ECV = Explained Common Variance. Omega = A model-based estimate of internal reliability of the multidimensional composite. Omega H (Hierarchical) = Percentage of variance in raw total scores that can be attributed to the individual differences on the general factor. Omega HS (Hierarchical Subscale) = Percentage of reliable variance of a subscale score after partitioning out variance attributed to the general factor. Relative Omega = Omega Hierarchical divided by Omega.

.69), along with high ECV (> .60; ours was .66) and high Omega Hierarchical (> .70; ours was .76) also means low risk of parameter bias. Hence, modeling the TAS-20 as a unidimensional instrument would not likely lead to significant measurement parameter bias (i.e., biased item factor loadings). There is also relative parameter bias – the difference between an item's loading in the unidimensional solution and its general factor loading in the bifactor model, divided by the general factor loading in the bifactor model. "Average parameter bias less than 10–15% is acceptable and poses no serious concern" (Rodriguez et al., 2016, p. 145). Our average relative parameter bias is within this range at 11.3%. Finally, there is explained common variance (ECV), which was .66 for the general factor and .80 for EOT, but only .19 and .20 for DIF and DDF, suggesting that DIF and DDF essentially remeasure the general factor.[4] In summary, the dimensional indices support the unidimensional structure of the TAS-20 (Table 4.2).

Reliability

Omega (ω) is a factor analytic model-based estimate of the internal reliability of the multidimensional composite scale. For the group factors, only those items that load on a factor are considered in the calculation, whereas for the general factor all items are taken into account. As can be seen in Table 4.2, the ω values range from .80 to .90 for the general factor and for DIF and DDF, indicating these factors are reliable; however, ω for EOT was only .59, replicating prior research that has found EOT to be unreliable. Omega Hierarchical (ωH) reflects the percentage of variance in raw total scores that can be attributed to the general factor, whereas Omega Hierarchical Subscale (ωHS) reflects the percentage of reliable variance of a subscale score after removing variance attributed to the general factor. Definitive guidelines for evaluating ωH and ωHS do not exist; however, Reise et al. (2013a) indicated that "tentatively, we can propose that a minimum would be greater than .50, and values closer to .75 would be much preferred" (p. 137). From this we can see that none of the group factors even met the .50 criterion, whereas the general factor met the .75 criteria.

Relative Omega (ωH/ω) is Omega Hierarchical or Omega Hierarchical Subscale divided by Omega. For the general factor this represents the percentage of reliable variance in the multidimensional composite that is due to the general factor; for the group factors, it represents the percentage of reliable variance in the subscale composite that is independent of the general factor. The relative ω for the general factor was .86, indicating that 86% of the reliable variance in the TAS-20 total scale score was due to the general factor. Thus, model-based reliability estimates support the use of the raw TAS-20 total score to represent general alexithymia. The relative ω for the group factors were DIF 16%, DDF 20%, and EOT 79% in terms of the proportion of the variance of the items loading on their factors that was independent of the general factor, indicating that (with the exception of EOT) the group factors largely remeasure the general factor.

Thus, the analysis of model-based dimensionality and reliability coefficients support the unidimensionality of the TAS-20 and therefore support the use of the raw total scale score, which can be said to represent the general alexithymia construct, supporting hypothesis H1. Given the evidence for the scale's unidimensionality and for the reliability of the general factor but not for the subscales, we recommend that only the total raw scale score be used in research and in clinical practice.

Descriptive Statistics

Raw-score-based correlation coefficients, alpha coefficients, means, and standard deviations for the TAS-20, NMAS, RAAS subscales, and the BAS are presented in Table 4.3.

Convergent and Concurrent Evidence for the Validity of the TAS-20

Based on the Chen et al. (2006) guidelines, we assessed the convergent and concurrent evidence for the unidimensional TAS-20's validity. In this model, latent factors for all scales were created using parcels as discussed above. A latent factor representing the general alexithymia factor was regressed on latent factors representing the validity measures of the NMAS, the 3 RAAS subscales, and the BAS. The CFA of the measurement model produced good fit to the data, χ^2 (174) = 554.58, $p < .001$, CFI = .961, TLI = .953, RMSEA = .056 (90% CI = .049, .062), SRMR = .04. All parcels had significant loadings of at least .40 on their respective factors. Next, regression paths were added from each of the

TABLE 4.3 Zero-order Correlations, Means, Standard Deviations, and Coefficient Alphas of Study Variables Raw Scores for Men

Variable	1	2	3	4	5	6	Mean	SD	Alpha
1. TAS-20	—						2.35	.78	.89
2. NMAS	.53**	—					3.91	1.08	.92
3. RAAS-Close	-.15**	-.62**	—				3.24	.83	.82
4. RAAS-Depend	-.28**	-.55**	.71**	—			3.03	.83	.81
5. RAAS-Anxiety	.34**	.38**	-.50**	-.62**	—		2.37	1.02	.92
6. BAS	-.21**	-.31**	.26**	-.23**	-.30**	—	42.87	10.73	.94

Note. $N = 505$. TAS-20 = Toronto Alexithymia Scale-20 (scores ranged from 1 to 5); NMAS = Normative Male Alexithymia Scale (scores ranged from 1 to 6.9); BAS = Body Attitudes Scale (scores ranged from 13 to 65); RAAS-Close = the Close subscale of the Revised Adult Attachment Scale (scores ranged from 1 to 5); RAAS-Depend = the Depend subscale of the Revised Adult Attachment Scale (scores ranged from 1 to 5); RAAS-Anxiety = the Anxiety subscale of the Revised Adult Attachment Scale (scores ranged from 1 to 5). $**p < .01$.

validity factors to the TAS-20 factor. The fit statistics for this model were identical to the measurement model, and thus also showed good fit. With regard to the validity hypotheses, Hypothesis **H2**, predicting that the TAS-20 will show a significant moderate coefficient when it is regressed on the latent factor of the NMAS, was supported ($B = 0.46$, $SE = .07$, 90% CI [.32, .60]; $\beta = .75$, $p < .001$, 95% CI [.53, .97]), providing convergent construct evidence for the validity of the TAS-20. Hypothesis **H3**, which stated that the TAS-20 will show a significant small negative coefficient when it is regressed on the latent factor of RAAS-Close subscale was not supported ($B = .17$, $SE = .23$, 95 % CI [–.28, .62]; $\beta = .16$, $p = .47$; 90% CI [–.28, .59]). Hypothesis **H4**, predicting that the TAS-20 will show a significant small negative coefficient when it is regressed on the latent factor of RAAS-Depend subscale was not supported ($B = .13$, $SE = .14$, 90% CI [–.13, .40]; $\beta = .16$, $p = .326$, 90% CI [–.16, .49]). Hypothesis **H5**, predicting that the TAS-20 will show a significant small positive coefficient when it is regressed on the latent factor of RAAS-Anxiety subscale was supported ($B = .20$, $SE = .04$, 90% CI [.12, .28], $\beta = .31$, $p < .001$, 90% CI [.19, .43]), providing concurrent criterion-related evidence for validity. Finally, Hypothesis **H6**, predicting that the TAS-20 will show a significant small-moderate negative coefficient when it is regressed on the latent factor of BAS was not supported ($B = –.02$, $SE = .04$, 90% CI [–.09, .05], $\beta = –.02$, $p = .615$, 90% CI [–.12, .07]). Thus, two out of five validity hypotheses were supported, one providing convergent evidence, and one providing criterion evidence.

Assessment of Measurement Invariance by Gender

Prior to conducting invariance analyses, we tested the fit of the unidimensional TAS-20 in separate analyses for men and women. To identify the model in the single- and multi-group CFA's, we constrained the latent factor variance to 1 and the mean to 0. Given that the unidimensional model did not fit the data well for the whole sample, it is not surprising that it also did not fit well for the unisex samples. For men, χ^2 (df) = 2100.44 (170), $p < .0001$, CFI = .543; TLI = .489; RMSEA = .133 (90% CI = .128, .138); SRMR = .106. For women, χ^2 (df) = 917.25 (170), $p < .0001$, CFI = .545, TLI = .492, RMSEA = .137 (90% CI = .128, .146), SRMR = 0.108. However, given the limitations we are working under (in terms of not being able to trim the model to improve fit), we proceeded to assess for invariance between genders by fitting multi-group CFA's to assess for configural, metric, and scalar invariance. The results are shown in Table 4.4. Comparing the configural to the metric invariance model, although the $\Delta\chi2$ was statistically significant, the ΔCFI was .007, under the cutoff of .01, thus supporting metric invariance. However, comparing the metric to the scalar model, the $\Delta\chi2$ was statistically significant and the ΔCFI was .012, over the cutoff of .01; hence scalar invariance failed.

TABLE 4.4 Model Fit Statistics and Comparisons of Nested Multiple Gender Group Models of the TAS-20

Invariance Model	χ^2 (df)	CFI, TLI	RMSEA [90% CI]	SRMR	BIC
Configural	1695.23 (340)	0.746, 0.716	0.093 [0.089, 0.098]	0.088	53,558.88
Metric	1750.52 (359)	0.739, 0.724	0.092 [0.088, 0.096]	0.097	53,481.85
Scalar	1834.99 (379)	0.727, 0.727	0.092 [0.088, 0.096]	0.099	53,428.79
Model Comparison:	$\Delta\chi^2$ (df)	p	ΔCFI	Conclusion	
Config. vs. Metric	50.95 (19)	<.001	0.007	Prefer metric, metric invariance supported.	
Metric vs. Scalar	81.90 (20)	<.001	0.012	Significant fit degradation, reject scalar invariance.	

DISCUSSION

The purpose of this study was to assess the evidence for using the total scale score of the Toronto Alexithymia Scale-20. Common factors, bifactor, hierarchical and unidimensional models were estimated, and none met contemporary standards for good fit. However, the analysis of model-based dimensionality and reliability coefficients supported the unidimensionality of the raw TAS-20 total score, which can be said to represent the general alexithymia construct. Convergent and concurrent evidence for validity was found in men using latent variables. It is an important reminder that assessing validity using latent variables is a more stringent approach than using raw scores, because it allows for the separation out of most sources of error. For example, in the present study, the raw score correlations of the TAS-20 with the five validity variables were all significant; yet only two regression coefficients were significant using the latent variable approach. Finally, the assessment of measurement invariance by gender supported metric invariance, indicating that cisgender men and women understand the scale in the same way, including the meaning of the scale scores and the distance between the scores.

Although evidence was found for modeling the TAS-20 as a unidimensional scale, and thus for the use of the total scale score, it should be noted that the fit of the unidimensional model is not optimal. We thus recommend, first, that researchers and clinicians use only the total scale score and not the subscales, and second, that the TAS-20 scale developers follow recommended procedures to trim composite measurement scales (c.f. Goetz et al., 2013) in order to improve the psychometric properties of the TAS-20 and in particular the fit to the data. While we were awaiting an editorial decision on this manuscript, we became aware that the TAS-20 scale developers had very recently published an article online in which they too recommended treating the TAS-20 as a unidimensional scale:

In general, our findings were consistent with previous studies indicating that TAS-20 total scores can be considered indicative of a single construct. The replication of these earlier results from previous investigations provides additional support for the use of a total TAS-20 score and questions the utility of using TAS-20 subscale scores. Based on these results, we recommend that researchers and clinicians use a single total TAS-20 score and not subscale scores (Carnovale, 2021, p. 1).

We wish to acknowledge some limitations of the current study. First, this was a cross-sectional study using self-report measures. The self-report nature of the surveys introduces the possibility that respondents approached the measures in a manner that make them look more socially desirable than they are (socially desirable responding/SDR). SDR was not measured in our study; however, SDR is not always a problem. As Tracey (2016, p. 229) put it:

> Perhaps the biggest recommendation is for researchers not to implicitly assume that SDR is harmful bias. There is an extensive literature that indicates that across many domains of psychology there is no strong support for such a view …

Second, we did not assess discriminant, predictive, and incremental evidence for validity, and test-retest evidence for reliability, which would be important tasks for future research. Third, our samples were collected from community and undergraduate participant pool subjects who self-selected to participate in this study. Recruitment via the internet or university classes also excluded potential participants of lower socioeconomic status. Further, there is less representation from communities of color with online samples. In addition, there were no transgender or non-binary people in our sample. We know from prior research that an intensive effort, including partnering with LGBTQI groups, is necessary to do this, and it should be done in future research. In effect, although participants were diverse in terms of age, they were predominantly White, Christian, educated beyond high school, cisgender, and heterosexual. Our results may thus not be representative of the general population and important differences may emerge with other samples. Additional research is certainly needed, especially work using more sophisticated sampling procedures to gather a representative sample of the United States population.

In conclusion, there is evidence for the use of the total raw (i.e., observed) scale score but not that of the subscales of the TAS-20 in both research and practice, which is important because of prior work that allowed for the establishment of criteria for diagnosing alexithymia (Taylor et al., 1988). However, in keeping with idea of "hidden invalidity" of psychological scales (Hussey & Hughes, 2020), the fit of the TAS-20 modeled as a unidimensional scale is suboptimal, and because of the poor fit to the data (replicating most studies on the TAS-20).

NOTES

2. Although the title references only 18 models, there was also a 19th model labeled "bifactor with negatively worded items dropped."
3. Although the sex question included the response options "transgender" and "other – please specify," none of the participants selected either of these options.
4. It should be noted, in terms of potential scale trimming, that the item ECV scores for the four of the five reverse-scored items were miniscule (the largest was .009), and two of them had elevated absolute relative parameter bias scores.

REFERENCES

Avalos, L., Tylka, T. L., & Wood-Barcalow, N. (2005). The body appreciation scale: Development and psychometric evaluation. *Body Image, 2*, 285–297. https://doi .org/10.1016/j.bodyim.2005.06.002

Bagby, R. M., Parker, J. D., & Taylor, G. J. (1994). The 20-item Toronto Alexithymia Scale: I. Item selection and cross validation of the factor structure. *Journal of Psychosomatic Research, 38*, 23–32. https://doi.org/10.1016/0022 -3999(94)90005-1

Carnovale, M., Taylor, G. J., Parker, J. D. A., Sanches, M., & Bagby, R. M. (2021, April 1). A bifactor analysis of the 20-Item Toronto Alexithymia Scale: Further support for a general alexithymia factor. *Psychological Assessment*. Advance online publication. http://dx.doi.org/10.1037/pas0001000

Chen, F. F. (2007). Sensitivity of goodness-of-fit indexes to lack of measurement invariance. *Structural Equation Modeling, 14*, 464–504. https://doi.org/10.1080 /10705510701301834

Chen, F. F., West, S. G., & Sousa, K. H. (2006). A comparison of bifactor and second-order models of quality of life. *Multivariate Behavioral Research, 41*, 189–225. https://doi.org/10.1207/s15327906mbr4102_5

Cheung, G. W., & Lau, R. S. (2012). A direct comparison approach for testing measurement invariance. *Organizational Research Methods, 15*, 167–198. https://doi.org/10.1177/1094428111421987

Cheung, G. W., & Rensvold, R. B. (2002). Evaluating goodness-of-fit indexes for testing measurement invariance. *Structural Equation Modeling, 9*, 233–255. https://doi.org/10.1207/S15328007SEM0902_5

Collins, N. L. (1996). Working models of attachment: Implications for explanation, emotion, and behavior. *Journal of Personality and Social Psychology, 71*, 810–832. https://doi.org/10.1037/0022-3514.71.4.810

Collins, N. L., & Read, S. J. (1990). Adult attachment, working models, and relationship quality in dating couples. *Journal of Personality and Social Psychology, 58*, 644–663. https://doi.org/10.1037/0022-3514.58.4.644

Dueber, D. M. (2017). Bifactor indices calculator: A microsoft excel-based tool to calculate various indices relevant to bifactor CFA models. https://doi.org/10 .13023/edp.tool.01. Retrieved from http://sites.education.uky.edu/apslab/ resources

Eng, W., Heimberg, R. G., Hart, T. A., Schneier, F. R., & Liebowitz, M. R. (2001). Attachment in individuals with social anxiety disorder: The relationship among adult attachment styles, social anxiety, and depression. *Emotion, 1*, 365–380. https://doi.org/10.1037/1528-3542.1.4.365

Erni, T., Lotscher, K., & Modestin, J. (1997). Two-factor solution of the 20-item Toronto Alexithymia Scale confirmed. *Psychopathology, 30*, 335–340. https://doi.org/10.1159/000285079

Ferguson, C. J. (2009). An effect size primer: A guide for clinicians and researchers. *Professional Psychology: Research and Practice, 40*, 532–538. https://doi.org/10.1037/a0015808

Gignac, G. E., Palmer, B. R., & Stough, C. (2007). A confirmatory factor analytic investigation of the TAS-20: Corroboration of a five-factor model and suggestions for improvement. *Journal of Personality Assessment, 89*, 247–257. https://doi.org/10.1080/00223890701629730

Goetz, C., Coste, J., Lemetayer, F., Rat, A., Montel, S., Recchia, S., Debouverie, M., Pouchot, J., Spitz, E., & Guillemin, F. (2013). Item reduction based on rigorous methodological guidelines is necessary to maintain validity when shortening composite measurement scales. *Journal of Clinical Epidemiology, 66*, 710–718. https://doi.org/10.1016/j.jclinepi.2012.12.015

Haviland, M. G., & Reise, S. P. (1996). Structure of the twenty-item Toronto Alexithymia Scale. *Journal of Personality Assessment, 66*, 116–125. https://doi.org/10.1207/s15327752jpa6601_9

Hu, L., & Bentler, P. M. (1998). Fit indices in covariance structure modeling: Sensitivity to underparameterized model misspecification. *Psychological Methods, 3*, 424–453. https://doi.org/10.1037/1082-989X.3.4.424

Humphreys, T. P., Wood, L. M., & Parker, J. D. A. (2009). Alexithymia and satisfaction in intimate relationships. *Personality and Individual Differences, 46*, 43–47. https://doi.org/10.1016/j.paid.2008.09.002

Hussey, I., & Hughes, S. (2020). Hidden invalidity among 15 commonly used measures in social and personality psychology. *Advances in Methods and Practices in Psychological Science*, 1–19. https://doi.org/10.1177/2515245919882903

Kahn, J. H. (2006). Factor analysis in counseling psychology research, training, and practice: Principles, advances, and applications. *The Counseling Psychologist, 34*, 684–718. https://doi.org/10.1177/0011000006286347

Karakis, E. N., & Levant, R. F. (2012). Is normative male alexithymia associated with relationship satisfaction, fear of intimacy and communication quality among men in heterosexual relationships. *Journal of Men's Studies, 20*, 179–186. https://doi.org/10.3149/jms.2003.179

Kline, R. B. (2016). *Principles and practice of structural equation modeling* (4th ed.). New York: Guilford.

Kooimana, C. G., Spinhovena, P., & Trijsburgc, R. W. (2002). The assessment of alexithymia: A critical review of the literature and a psychometric study of the Toronto Alexithymia Scale-20. *Journal of Psychosomatic Research, 53*, 1083–1090. https://doi.org/10.4236/psych.2012.33032

Leone, J. E., Wise, K. A., Mullin, E. M., Harmon, W., Moreno, N., & Drewniany, J. (2015). The effects of pubertal timing and alexithymia on symptoms of muscle dysmorphia and the drive for muscularity in men. *Psychology of Men & Masculinity, 16*, 67–77. https://doi.org/10.1037/a0035920

Levant, R. F., Allen, P. A., & Lien, M.-C. (2014). Alexithymia in men: How and when does the deficit in the processing of emotions occur? *Psychology of Men and Masculinity, 15*, 324–334. https://doi.org/10.1037/a0033860

Levant, R. F., Good, G. E., Cook, S., O'Neil, J., Smalley, K. B., Owen, K. A., & Richmond, K. (2006). The normative male alexithymia scale: Measurement of a gender-linked syndrome. *Psychology of Men and Masculinity, 7*, 212–224. https://doi.org/10.1037/1524-9220.7.4.212

Loas, G., Braun, S., Linkowski, P., & Luminet, O. (2015). Determination of the cutoff threshold on the Bermond-Vorst Alexithymia Questionnaire–20 form B: A study of 560 young adults. *Psychological Reports, 117*(3), 1–9. https://doi.org/10.2466 /03.PR0.117c24z2. ISSN 0033-2941

Loas, G., Otmani, O., Verrier, A., Fremaux, D., & Marchand, M. P. (1996). Factor analysis of the French version of the 20-item Toronto Alexithymia Scale (TAS-20). *Psychopathology, 29*, 139–144. https://doi.org/10.1159/000284983

Meganck, R., Vanheule, S., & Desmet, M. (2008). Factorial validity and measurement invariance of the 20-item Toronto Alexithymia Scale in clinical and non-clinical samples. *Assessment, 15*, 36–47. https://doi.org/10.1177/1073191107306140

Muthén, L. K., & Muthén, B. O. (1998–2015). *Mplus user's guide* (7th ed.). Los Angeles: Muthén & Muthén.

Parent, M. C., & Bradstreet, T. C. (2019). The strong, silent type(ology): Examining intersections of alexithymia and the drive for muscularity. *Journal of Men's Studies, 27*, 66–88. https://doi.org/10.1177/1060826518782976

Parker, J. A., Bagby, R. M., Taylor, G. J., Endler, N. S., & Schmitz, P. (1993). Factorial validity of the 20-item Toronto Alexithymia Scale. *European Journal of Personality, 7*, 221–232. Retrieved from ebscohost.com. https://doi.org/10.1002 /per.2410070403

Parker, J. A., Taylor, G. J., & Bagby, M. J. (2003). The 20-item Toronto Alexithymia Scale III. Reliability and factorial validity in a community population. *Journal of Psychosomatic Research, 55*, 269–275. https://doi.org/10.1016/S0022 -3999(02)00578-0

Preece, D., Becerra, R., Allan, A., Robinson, K., & Dandy, J. (2017). Establishing the theoretical components of alexithymia via factor analysis: Introduction and validation of the attention-appraisal model of alexithymia. *Personality and Individual Differences, 119*, 341–352. https://doi.org/10.1016/j.paid.2017.08.003

Ravitz, P., Maunder, R., Hunter, J., Sthankiya, B., & Lancee, W. (2010). Adult attachment measures: A 25-year review. *Journal of Psychosomatic Research, 69*, 419–432. https://doi.org/10.1016/j.jpsychores.2009.08.006

Reise, S. P., Bonifay, W. E., & Haviland, M. G. (2013a). Scoring and modeling psychological measures in the presence of multidimensionality. *Journal of Personality Assessment, 95*, 129–140. https://doi.org/10.1080/00223891.2012 .725437

Reise, S. P., Scheines, R., Widaman, K. F., & Haviland, M. G. (2013b). Multidimensionality and structural coefficient bias in structural equation modeling a bifactor perspective. *Educational and Psychological Measurement, 73,* 5–26. https://doi.org/10.1177/0013164412449831

Ritz, T., & Kannapin, O. (2000). The construct validity of a German Version of the Toronto Alexithymia Scale. *Zeitschrift Für Differentielle und Diagnostische Psychologie, 21,* 49–64. https://doi.org/10.1024//0170-1789.21.1.49

Rodriguez, A., Reise, S. P., & Haviland, M. G. (2016). Evaluating bifactor models: Calculating and interpreting statistical indices. *Psychological Methods, 21,* 137–150. https://doi.org/10.1037/met0000045

Russell, D. W., Kahn, J. H., Spoth, R., & Altmaier, E. M. (1998). Analyzing data from experimental studies: A latent variable structural equation modeling approach. *Journal of Counseling Psychology, 45,* 18–29. https://doi.org/10.1037/0022 -0167.45.1.18

Satorra, A., & Bentler, P. M. (1999). *A scaled difference chi-square test statistic for moment structure analysis* (UCLA Statistics Series #260). Los Angeles: University of California.

Soper, D. (2013). *A priori sample size calculator for structural equation models [Computer software].* Retrieved July 2, 2016, from http://www.danielsoper.com/ statcalc/calculator.aspx?id=89

Taylor, G. H., Bagby, R. M., Ryan, D. P., Parker, J. D. A., Doody, F. F., & Keefe, P. (1988). Criterion validity of the Toronto Alexithymia Scale. *Psychosomatic Medicine, 50,* 500–509. https://doi.org/10.1097/00006842-198809000-00006

Taylor, G. J. (2004). Alexithymia: Twenty-five years of theory and research. In I. Nyklicek, L. Temoshok, & A. Vingerhoets (Eds.), *Emotional expression and health: Advances in theory, assessment and clinical applications* (pp. 137–153). New York: Brunner-Routledge.

Taylor, G. J., Parker, J. D., Bagby, R. M., & Acklin, M. W. (1992). Alexithymia and somatic complaints in psychiatric out-patients. *Journal of Psychosomatic Research, 36,* 417–424. https://doi.org/10.1016/0022-3999(92)90002-J

Tracey, T. J. G. (2016). A note on socially desirable responding. *Journal of Counseling Psychology, 63,* 224–232. https://doi.org/10.1037/cou0000135

Tuliao, A. P., Klanecky, A. K., Landoy, B. V. N., & McChargue, D. E. (2019). Toronto Alexithymia Scale–20: Examining 18 competing factor structure solutions in a US sample and a Philippines sample. *Assessment, 27.* Advance online publication. https://doi.org/10731911188824030

Tylka, T. L. (2013). Evidence for the body appreciation scale's measurement equivalence/invariance between U.S. College women and men. *Body Image, 10,* 415–418. https://doi.org/10.1016/j.bodyim.2013.02.006

The Normative Male Alexithymia Scale: Measurement of a Gender-Linked Syndrome[1]

Ronald F. Levant, Glenn E. Good, Stephen W. Cook, James M. O'Neil, K. Bryant Smalley, Karen Owen, and Katherine Richmond

STUDY 1

Method

Participants and Procedures

The sample for the examination of the factor structure for NMAS items consisted of 266 men enrolled in introductory psychology classes at a large public university in the south-central United States. The majority of participants were between 18 and 22 years old ($n = 248$; 93%) and described their ethnicity as White (non-Hispanic) ($n = 222$; 84%). More specific demographic information about this sample was unavailable since the data were collected as part of an optional survey of all consenting introductory psychology students. Participation in the survey served as one option for students to satisfy course requirements. General consent and debriefing forms were used. Participants completed the 29 items initially developed for the Normative Male Alexithymia Scale (NMAS), in addition to several other measures for other research studies.

The Normative Male Alexithymia Scale (Levant et al., 2004) was designed to assess Normative Male Alexithymia. Respondents indicate their responses to questions about their experience of emotions using a Likert-type format (1 = *strongly disagree*, 7 = *strongly agree*). For the total scale score, after recoding reverse-worded items, scores are averaged, with a higher score indicating greater Normative Male Alexithymia. Based on published descriptions of the

DOI: 10.4324/9781003378518-7

Normative Male Alexithymia construct (Levant, 1992, 1995, 1998), senior scholars with particular expertise in the content area generated 15 items. Fourteen additional items reflecting aspects of the normative alexithymia construct were adapted or borrowed (with authors' permission) from instruments designed to tap related constructs: The Gender Role Conflict Scale (O'Neil et al., 1986); the Emotional Openness Scale (Komiya, 2000); the Toronto Alexithymia Scale-20; and the Masculine Gender Role Stress Scale (Eisler & Skidmore, 1987). The final pool of 29 items was then reviewed by other masculinity scholars who confirmed that the items tapped the normative alexithymia construct. (See Appendix for the listing of the original 29 items and their sources.)

Results

Exploratory factor analysis was used to extract the latent factors underlying the NMAS items. While six factors had eigenvalues greater than 1.00, the scree test more strongly supported one-, two-, or three-factor solutions (with 32%, 40%, and 45% of the total variance accounted for by these factors, respectively). We examined these factor solutions, considering both varimax (orthogonal) and oblimin (oblique) rotations. The one-factor solution utilizing a factor loading criterion of .40 was preferable in terms of both statistical and conceptual clarity (factor loadings are included with items in the Appendix). The 20 items which loaded on this factor are identical to those that emerged when conducting a one-factor principal components analysis (again with item factor loadings > .40). Coefficient alpha was .93 in this sample indicating excellent internal consistency for the 20-item scale.

STUDY 2

Consistent with Levant's theory of Normative Male Alexithymia, we hypothesized that men's scores on the Normative Male Alexithymia Scale would correlate positively with: (a) alexithymia (i.e., TAS-20 scores), (b) traditional masculinity ideology (i.e., Male Role Norms Inventory total scores), and (c) the restricted emotionality aspect of traditional masculinity ideology (i.e., Restricted Emotionality subscale scores of the Male Role Norms Inventory). Similarly, we hypothesized that (d) men would score higher than women on the Normative Male Alexithymia Scale (given men's emotion-related experiences with masculine socialization). Based on our review of the literature on sex differences on the TAS-20 in non-clinical samples, we also hypothesized that (e) in our non-clinical sample, men would score higher than women on the TAS-20. Finally (f), we examined whether men's NMAS scores significantly predicted their MRNI scores above and beyond that predicted by their TAS-20 scores, as evidence for incremental validity.

Method

Participants and Procedures

Participants were recruited from undergraduate introductory psychology courses at the same south-central public university as in Study 1. A total of 407 students (192 men, 210 women, and five who declined to identify their sex) participated, with 91% being between 17 and 20, 8% between 21 and 24, and 1% between 25 and 45 years old. The ethnicity/race composition of the sample was: Caucasian = 331 (81%); Latino/Latina = 41 (10%); African American = 10 (3%); Asian American = 10 (3%); Other = 9 (2%); Missing = 6 (2%). Sexual orientation was measured on a scale of 1 (attracted exclusively to the same sex) to 7 (attracted exclusively to the other sex). Of the sample of 407 students, 3% ($n = 14$) identified themselves as exclusively attracted to the same sex, 6% of students ($n = 25$) identified themselves between the two ends of the continuum, and 89% ($n = 363$) identified themselves as exclusively attracted to the other sex. Married students comprised 4% ($n = 16$) of the sample, single students 56% ($n = 229$), divorced students .5% ($n = 2$), and "seriously dating" students comprised 38% ($n = 155$). More than 60% of the sample (64%, $n = 260$) reported family income of more than $60,000, and 90% ($n = 368$) identified themselves as middle, upper middle, or upper class.

Some participants completed the NMAS for both Study 1 and Study 2. Sixty-five of these participants (29 men and 36 women) provided permission to compare their NMAS scores in both studies in order to provide data about test-retest reliability. This sub-sample of participants was predominantly Caucasian (87%), ranged between 17 and 45 years old (mode = 19 years), reported mostly an exclusive attraction to the opposite gender (91%), and identified mostly being either "single" (57%) or "seriously dating" (40%), and being middle (48%) or upper middle class (48%).

Participants completed the NMAS, MRNI, TAS-20, and a brief demographic questionnaire. Participation is this study was one option to fulfill a course requirement, with all aspects of the study complying with campus IRB procedures (e.g., informed consent, right to withdraw, and debriefing).

Measures

Normative Male Alexithymia Scale (NMAS). Information on the NMAS (Levant et al., 2004) is provided in Study 1.

Toronto Alexithymia Scale (TAS-20). The TAS-20 (Bagby, Parker et al., 1994; Bagby, Taylor et al., 1994) is a 20-item inventory designed to assess clinical alexithymia. Sample items include, "I am often puzzled by sensations in my body," and "I don't know what's going on inside me." Participants indicate the extent of their agreement/disagreement on a five-point Likert-type scale, with higher scores indicating greater alexithymia. The instrument was derived from a factor analysis of a longer version of the scale (Bagby, Parker et al., 1994; Bagby, Taylor et al., 1994; Taylor, 1994). The TAS-20 scale score was derived by averaging individual item scores. Internal consistency in the present study was good (α = .84 for men and .86 for women).

Male Role Norms Inventory (MRNI). The Male Role Norms Inventory (Levant et al., 1992) was developed to measure the endorsement of both traditional and non-traditional masculinity ideology. The original MRNI is a 57-item scale consisting of statements to which respondents indicate their degree of agreement/disagreement on a seven-point Likert-type scale. Data supporting the divergent and convergent construct validity of the MRNI were reported by Levant and Fischer (1998). For this study, we used the abbreviated 49-item version of the MRNI (MRNI-49; Berger et al., 2005), which focuses solely on traditional masculinity ideology. Sample items include, "Being a little down in the dumps is not a good reason for a man to act depressed" and "Men should be detached in emotionally charged situations." The MRNI Total and Restrictive Emotionality subscale scores were derived by averaging individual item scores. Coefficient alphas were good (α = .96 for MRNI total scale, and .85 for MRNI Restrictive Emotionality subscale).

Results

A confirmatory factor analysis was conducted to determine if the 20-item, one-factor NMAS structure identified in Study 1 was replicated by the data for male participants (*n* = 186) in this study. Utilizing maximum likelihood confirmatory factor analysis with robust statistics on the covariance matrixes and specifying the variance for the one factor to be fixed at 1.0, no problems were encountered in deriving the solution. As typically found using confirmatory factor analysis of this type, the chi-square was statistically significant (Sartorra-Bentler scaled chi-square = 368; *df* = 170; *p* < .0001). Other fit indices provided only modest support for the 20-item, one-factor structure (i.e., non-normed or Tucker-Lewis fit index [NNFI] = .85; comparative fit index [CFI] = .87; root mean-square error of approximation [RMSEA] = .08). Further, an exploratory principal factor analysis in this sample replicated the findings that the same 20 items found in Study 1 loaded on a single factor (when item factor loadings greater than .40 were considered). Therefore, the 20-item, one-factor NMAS solution , while not ideal, was determined to be the optimal factor solution and was retained for all subsequent analyses in this study.

Internal consistency was excellent, with coefficient alphas of .92 for men and .93 for women for NMAS scores. Test–retest analyses indicated strong support for the temporal stability of the NMAS; specifically, test-retest correlations for the

NMAS total scores were .91 for men ($n = 29$) and .86 for women ($n = 36$) over a one- to two-month period.

Correlations, means, standard deviations, ranges, and coefficient alphas for all variables for men only are presented in Table 5.1. Means for the MRNI and TAS-20 are similar to those found in other published research with college men (e.g., Levant et al., 2003; Fischer & Good, 1997, respectively). The 20-item, one-factor NMAS was found to correlate significantly, as predicted, with the TAS-20 ($r = .72$), MRNI (total scale score; $r = .35$), and MRNI Restricted Emotionality subscale ($r = .50$) among male participants. Hence, in male participants, greater self-reported Normative Male Alexithymia is associated with greater clinical alexithymia, greater endorsement of total traditional masculinity ideology, and greater endorsement of the traditional masculine norm of restricted emotionality. ANOVAs were conducted to investigate potential sex differences on all three instruments. As shown in Table 5.2, in accord with our hypotheses, men scored significantly higher than women on the NMAS ($p < .0001$) and TAS-20 ($p < .001$).

Hierarchical multiple regressions were computed to examine whether the NMAS scores significantly predicted MRNI Total and Restrictive Emotional scores beyond that predicted by TAS-20 scores (see Table 5.3). As anticipated from the correlation results, TAS-20 scores significantly predicted MRNI Total and Restrictive Emotionality scores in the first step of the regressions. When NMAS scores were entered in the next step, they added significantly to the prediction of both MRNI Total and Restrictive Emotionality scores (p's > .05). Additionally, after NMAS scores were entered into the regression TAS-20 scores no longer significantly predicted MRNI Total or Restrictive Emotionality

TABLE 5.1 Correlations, Means, Standard Deviations, Ranges and Coefficient Alphas for Men on the TAS-20, MRNI, and NMAS

Variable	TAS-20	MRNI	MRNI REM	NMAS
TAS-20				
MRNI	.34*			
MRNI REM	.42*	.83*		
NMAS	.72*	.35*	.50*	
Mean	2.50	4.20	3.60	3.60
SD	.54	.86	1.04	1.03
Range	1.05–3.65	1.47–6.31	1.0–6.57	1.20–6.00
α	.84	.96	.85	.92
n	188	183	191	186

Note. TAS-20 = Toronto Alexithymia Scale-20; MRNI = Masculine Role Norms Inventory total score; MRNI REM = Restricted Emotionality subscale of the Masculine Role Norms Inventory; NMAS = Normative Masculine Alexithymia Scale.
*$p < .01$.

TABLE 5.2 Gender Differences on the NMAS and TAS-20

Instrument/Gender	n	M	SD	F	p
NMAS					
Men	186	3.60	1.03	37.7	.0001
Women	203	2.96	1.03		
TAS-20					
Men	188	2.50	.54	11.2	.001
Women	206	2.31	.58		

Note. NMAS = Normative Masculine Alexithymia Scale; TAS-20 = Toronto Alexithymia Scale-20.

TABLE 5.3 Summary of Hierarchical Regression Analysis for Alexithymia and Normative Male Alexithymia Predicting Male Role Norms

Variable	B	SE B	β	F	R^2
Traditional Masculinity Ideology (n = 173)					
Step 1				21.08*	.11
Alexithymia	0.53	0.12	0.33*		
Step 2				13.00*	.13
Alexithymia	0.27	0.17	0.17		
Normative Male Alexithymia	0.18	0.09	0.22*		
Restrictive Emotionality (n = 181)					
Step 1				37.88*	.17
Alexithymia	0.80	0.13	0.42*		
Step 2				30.31*	.25
Alexithymia	0.23	0.18	0.12		
Normative Male Alexithymia	0.41	0.09	0.41*		

Note. For Traditional Masculinity Ideology, ΔR^2 = .02 for Step 2 ($p\Delta R^2$ < .05). For Restrictive Emotionality, = .08 for Step 2 (p < .05)
*p < .05.

scores (p's > .05). Both measures of alexithymia (TAS-20 and NMAS) combined accounted for 13% of the variance of traditional masculinity ideology and 25% of the variance of restrictive emotionality as assessed by the MRNI. These regression results indicate that the NMAS contributes significantly above and beyond the TAS-20 to the prediction of masculinity ideology. (Table 5.3)

DISCUSSION

This investigation sought to provide an initial assessment of the psychometric properties of the Normative Male Alexithymia Scale, an instrument designed to assess sub-clinical aspects of difficulty recognizing and describing emotions theoretically linked to traditional masculine socialization. Findings provide strong evidence that scores on the NMAS were internally consistent and had very good test-retest reliability (temporal stability) over a one- to two-month period. Both exploratory and confirmatory factor analyses provided some, though not ideal, support for a one-factor structure, which should continue to be evaluated in future research. Evidence supporting the construct validity of the NMAS was provided by findings that scores on the NMAS were related to scores on the Toronto Alexithymia Scale and Male Role Norms Inventory (both total scale and Restricted Emotionality subscale). Hierarchical multiple regressions indicate that the NMAS contributes significantly above and beyond the TAS-20 to the prediction of masculinity ideology. Further, as hypothesized, in this non-clinical population, men scored higher than women on normative male alexithymia (as measured by the NMAS) and alexithymia (as measured by the Toronto Alexithymia Scale). These initial findings provide evidence supporting the psychometric properties of the NMAS in assessing Normative Male Alexithymia in non-clinical samples of men.

The current study is limited by the use of exclusively self-report data and a sample drawn from a single institution. It should also be noted that one item in the 20-item NMAS was adopted from the TAS-20, which likely slightly bolsters the correlation between these scales. Hence, additional studies of the psychometric properties of the NMAS are warranted.

The NMAS was designed to measure a mild form of alexithymia theorized to be normative for men. This theoretical formulation is based on research demonstrating that the requirement to restrict emotional expression is a central aspect of traditional masculine norms, and that boys are socialized to restrict the expression of emotions. Although we have found that men experience mild alexithymia more frequently than do women, that NMAS scores are correlated with the endorsement of traditional masculinity ideology (a construct theorized to be related to masculine socialization), and that the NMAS demonstrates incremental validity beyond that provided by current measures of clinical alexithymia (e.g., the TAS) in predicting the endorsement of traditional masculinity ideology, we have not demonstrated that these differences are due to socialization, and thus we have not tested the central element of the theory. We thus do not know whether the NMAS is related to masculine socialization. In order to say that the NMAS is related to masculine socialization, we would have to use a measure of masculine socialization, which currently does not exist. Hence, at this stage of instrument development this question cannot be fully answered.

Future researchers may want to investigate potential relations of sub-clinical alexithymia to other constructs of interest – including both clinical problems such as depression, substance abuse, psychosomatic illness, and relationship concerns and more subtle outcomes, such as men's lack of willingness to use mental health and medical services or engage in prevention and health promotion programs. Additionally, if evidence for the prevalence and harmful effects of Normative Male Alexithymia are detected, such findings may provide greater impetus for the development and evaluation of preventive and remedial interventions (e.g., Levant, 1998; Levant & Kelley, 1989; Levant & Kopecky, 1995; Mahalik et al., 2003; Robertson & Fitzgerald, 1992). These approaches appear promising in assisting boys and men in acquiring a vocabulary of emotions and in developing specific emotional skills sets needed to recognize and communicate emotions in themselves and others – skills termed "emotional competence" (Good, 1998).

In sum, this study provides encouraging information about the psychometric properties of the NMAS, the first scale designed to specifically assess Normative Male Alexithymia. This brief self-report instrument has potential value for both advancing research about mild (sub-clinical) alexithymia, and for providing practitioners and their male clients with an assessment tool for this potentially clinically relevant phenomenon.

APPENDIX

Normative Male Alexithymia Scale (NMAS) – Original Items

DIRECTIONS: Please use the scale below to indicate the extent to which you personally agree or disagree with each statement. There are no right or wrong responses.

1	2	3	4	5	6	7
Strongly Disagree	Disagree	Slightly Disagree	Neutral or Undecided	Slightly Agree	Agree	Strongly Agree

1. My romantic partner or spouse seems to know what I am feeling even when I don't. (–.23)
2. When someone lets me down I get very angry. (.10)
3. I don't think I am upset but then I get a headache, upset stomach or stiff neck and then I realize that I have been upset. (.18)
4. *If I am upset or worried I don't like to show it for fear that I will be seen as weak*. (.50)
5. *I feel comfortable expressing my affection to family members and friends*. (–.43)
6. *It does not usually occur to me to deal with my stress by talking about what is bothering me*. (.59)
7. *I find it is very hard to cry*. (.49)

8. *When asked, I can easily give an account of what I am feeling.* (−.64)
9. I am quite interested in my emotional life and spend a good deal of time mulling over what I am feeling. (−.23)
10. *I have no trouble putting my feelings into words and discussing them with others.* (−.67)
11. I often don't realize that I am getting angry until suddenly I blow up. (.23)
12. *When someone close to me hurts my feelings, I am able to tell them that I am hurt.* (−.59)
13. *I enjoy discussing my innermost feelings with my romantic partner, spouse, or best friend.* (−.59)
14. I am often confused about what emotion I am feeling. (.28)
15. When I am upset, I don't know if I am sad, frightened, or angry. (.31)
16. *It is difficult for me to reveal my innermost feelings, even to close friends.* (.72)
17. *If someone asks how I am feeling, I typically say what I am <u>not</u> feeling (e.g., "not too bad").* (.50)
18. *I don't see much value in talking about feelings.* (.61)
19. *I have difficulty telling others that I care about them.* (.66)
20. *I have difficulty expressing my emotional needs to my romantic partner, spouse, or best friend.* (.72)
21. *I have difficulty expressing my innermost feelings.* (.83)
22. *Talking about my feelings during sexual relations is difficult for me.* (.70)
23. *I do not like to show my emotions to other people.* (.79)
24. *It is too risky to express my emotions to other people.* (.68)
25. *I am comfortable telling someone that I am afraid of something.* (−.42)
26. I am comfortable talking with a friend who is upset. (−.28)
27. *I like my feelings.* (−.52)
28. By feeling a number of different emotions I am a more interesting person. (−.30)
29. *I don't like to talk with others about my feelings.* (.82)

Notes. Bold italicized items (those with factor loadings above .40) were retained in the 20-item scale. Numbers in parentheses indicate loading in a one-factor solution principal factor analysis ($N = 266$ men).

Scoring Instructions: To obtain the total score (mean item score), reverse the scoring of reverse-scored items, sum the responses, and divide by 20. Reverse-scored items = 5, 8, 9, 10, 12, 13, 25, 26, 27, and 28.

The following items were adopted with permission from the following instruments (* indicates that items were modified; **bold** indicates items retained in 20-item scale). Items #:

19, 20, 21*, 22*, 23, 24* from the Gender Role Conflict Scale (O'Neil et al., 1986).

27, 28, **29** from the Emotional Openness Scale (Komiya, 2000).

14, 15, **16** from the Toronto Alexithymia Scale-20 (Bagby, Parker et al., 1994; Bagby, Taylor et al., 1994).

25*, 26* from the Masculine Gender Role Stress Scale (Eisler & Skidmore, 1987).

NOTE

1. Chapter 5, entire chapter. Copyright © 2006 by the American Psychological Association. Reproduced and adapted with permission. The official citation that should be used in referencing this material is Levant, R. F., Good, G. E., Cook, S., O'Neil, J., Smalley, K. B., Owen, K. A., & Richmond, K. (2006). Validation of the normative male alexithymia scale: Measurement of a gender-linked syndrome. *Psychology of Men and Masculinity, 7,* 212–224. https://doi.org/10.1037/1524-9220.7.4.212 No further reproduction or distribution is permitted without written permission from the American Psychological Association.

REFERENCES

Bagby, R. M., Parker, J. D. A., & Taylor, G. J. (1994). The twenty-item Toronto Alexithymia Scale-I. Item selection and cross-validation of the factor structure. *Journal of Psychosomatic Research, 38,* 22–32. https://doi.org/10.1016/0022 -3999(94)90005-1

Bagby, R. M., Taylor, G. J., & Parker, J. D. A. (1994). The twenty-item Toronto Alexithymia Scale--II. Convergent, discriminant, and concurrent validity. *Journal of Psychosomatic Research, 38,* 33–40. https://doi.org/10.1016/0022 -3999(94)90006-X

Berger, J. M., Levant, R. F., McMillan, K. K., Kelleher, W., & Sellers, A. (2005). Impact of gender role conflict, traditional masculinity ideology, alexithymia, and age on men's attitudes toward psychological help seeking. *Psychology of Men and Masculinity, 6,* 73–78. https://doi.org/10.1037/1524-9220.6.1.73

Eisler, R. M., & Skidmore, J. R. (1987). Masculine gender role stress: Scale development and component factors in the appraisal of stressful situations. *Behavior Modification, 11,* 123–136. https://doi.org/10.1177/01454455870112001

Fischer, A. R., & Good, G. E. (1997). Men and psychotherapy: An investigation of alexithymia, intimacy, and masculine gender roles. *Psychotherapy, 34,* 160–170. https://doi.org/10.1037/h0087646

Good, G. E. (1998). Missing and underrepresented aspects of men's lives. *Society for the Psychological Study of Men and Masculinity Bulletin, 3*(2), 1–2. https://doi .org/10.1037/e411792005-001

Komiya, N. (2000). Development of the emotional openness scale. *Dissertation Abstracts International, 60*(12-B), 6417. (UMI No. AAI9953873).

Levant, R. F. (1992). Toward the reconstruction of masculinity. *Journal of Family Psychology, 5*, 379–402. https://doi.org/10.1037/0893-3200.5.3-4.379

Levant, R. F. (1995). Toward the reconstruction of masculinity. In R. Levant & W. S. Pollack (Eds.), *A new psychology of men* (pp. 229–251). New York: Basic Books.

Levant, R. F. (1998). Desperately seeking language: Understanding, assessing, and treating normative male alexithymia. In W. Pollack & R. Levant (Eds.), *New psychotherapy for men* (pp. 35–56). New York: John Wiley.

Levant, R. F., & Fischer, J. (1998). The male role norms inventory. In C. Davis, W. Yarber, R. Bauserman, G. Schreer, & S. Davis (Eds.), *Handbook of sexuality-related measures* (pp. 469–472). Thousand Oaks, CA: Sage.

Levant, R. F., Good, G., Cook, S., Richmond, K., Owen, K., & Smally, B. (2004, July). *Validation of the Normative Male Alexithymia* Scale (NMAS). Paper presented at the 112th Annual Convention of the American Psychological Association, Honolulu.

Levant, R. F., Hirsch, L., Celentano, E., Cozza, T. Hill, S., MacEachern, M., Marty, N., & Schnedeker, J. (1992). The male role: An investigation of contemporary norms. *Journal of Mental Health Counseling, 14*, 325–337.

Levant, R. F., & Kelly, J. (1989). *Between father and child: How to become the kind of father you want to be.* New York: Viking.

Levant, R. F., & Kopecky, G. (1995). *Masculinity reconstructed.* New York: Plume.

Levant, R. F., Richmond, K., Majors, R. G., Inclan, J. E., Rossello, J. M., Heesacker, M., et al. (2003). A multicultural investigation of masculinity ideology and alexithymia. *Psychology of Men and Masculinity, 4*, 91–99. https://doi.org/10.1037/1524-9220.4.2.91

Mahalik, J. R., Good, G. E., & Englar-Carlson, M. (2003). Masculinity scripts, presenting concerns and help-seeking: Implications for practice and training. *Professional Psychology: Theory, Research and Practice, 34*, 123–131. https://doi.org/10.1037/0735-7028.34.2.123

O'Neil, J. M., Helms, B., Gable, R. David, L. & Wrightsman, L. (1986). Gender-role conflict scale: College men's fear of femininity. *Sex Roles, 14*(5/6), 335–350. https://doi.org/10.1007/BF00287583

Robertson, J. M., & Fitzgerald, L. F. (1992). Overcoming the masculine mystique: Preferences for alternative forms of assistance among men who avoid counseling. *Journal of Counseling Psychology, 39*, 240–246. https://doi.org/10.1037/0022-0167.39.2.240

Taylor, G. J. (1994). The alexithymia construct: Conceptualization, validation, and relationship with basic dimensions of personality. *New Trends in Experimental and Clinical Psychiatry, 10*, 61–74.

CHAPTER SIX

The Development and Evaluation of a Brief Form of the Normative Male Alexithymia Scale (NMAS-BF)[1]

Ronald F. Levant and Mike C. Parent

INTRODUCTION

In the past 30 years, psychologists have made significant advancements in the measurement of masculinity-related constructs, such as gender role conflict (O'Neil, 2008), conformity to masculine norms (Mahalik et al., 2003) and masculinity ideology (Levant et al., 2013, 2016). The present chapter focuses on one such construct – Normative Male Alexithymia (NMA) and undertakes the development of a brief form of an extant scale designed to assess this construct with improved psychometric properties – the Normative Male Alexithymia Scale-Brief Form (NMAS-BF).

To assess some men's socialized limitations in emotional expression, Levant et al. (2006) developed the Normative Male Alexithymia Scale (NMAS). Exploratory and confirmatory factor analyses using separate samples indicated that the NMAS consisted of a single 20-item factor. Men's scores on the NMAS displayed very good internal consistency ($\alpha = .92$) and test-retest reliability ($r = .91$) over a one to two month period. Results of analyses of sex differences, relations of the NMAS with other instruments, and its incremental validity in predicting masculinity ideology provided evidence supporting the validity of the scale. However, the incremental fit indices did not support the factor structure of the original NMAS using contemporary standards (i.e., TLI = .85, CFI = .87). Although RMSEA (0.08) met the criterion of < .08, Gignac et al. (2007, p. 248) pointed out that such absolute fit indices "may erroneously suggest satisfactory levels of model fit simply because the items are only weakly correlated." Hence there is a need for measure with acceptable fit statistics. Furthermore, the

DOI: 10.4324/9781003378518-8

20-item NMAS is long for a unidimensional scale, potentially creating participant fatigue as the NMAS is likely to be one of several assessments used in batteries related to masculine socialization and emotional expression.

The Present Study

The present study was designed to extend prior work on the NMAS. There were four objectives. The first aim was to conduct another exploratory factor analysis (EFA) of the NMAS. There were several reasons for undertaking this EFA: It has been over ten years since the first one was conducted, the initial EFA was conducted with college students (Levant et al., 2006) whereas the present sample includes a wider range of ages in participants collected online, and the new EFA results will be used to develop a brief form of the NMAS (NMAS-BF). Based on prior literature, hypothesis 1 (**H1**) is advanced, that evidence will be found for one-factor dimensionality of the NMAS. The second aim was to develop candidate models of the NMAS-BF and to compare them using confirmatory factor analysis. Item selection in scale development is often guided by classical test theory (CTT), in which the highest-loading items from an EFA are chosen to compose the final scale, and one of the candidate models will be developed this way (i.e., the CTT model). However, several NMAS items have similar content. Such content overlap may result in strong correlations among these items and potentially suboptimal content overlap among the highest-loading items (i.e., that the items selected for the NMAS-BF, based solely on factor loading strength, could be redundant or assess a limited range of the construct of interest). Based on this anticipated challenge, we decided a priori that we would also select items based on a combination of item loading and an examination of content to reduce redundancy (i.e., an optimized CTT model). Finally, item response theory (IRT) has more recently been advocated as superior to CTT for item selection (DeVellis, 2016; Mallinckrodt et al., 2016). In using CTT for selection of items on a short form, one would select the highest-loading items for retention in the short form of the measure. In contrast, IRT, as applied to the development of measures such as the NMAS-BF, emphasizes item selection based on dispersing items across degrees of "difficulty" (for a Likert-type scale, difficulty reflects whether an item tends to be endorsed or not endorsed). Paradoxically, because items selected via IRT are likely to assess a wider range of the construct of interest than those selected by CCT, the items are likely to be less correlated and the model fit for an IRT-derived model would be superior to a CTT-derived model while assessing a broader range of the construct than the CTT-derived items. The objective was thus to generate three candidate models of the NMAS-BF: One based on CTT (Model 1), one based on CTT optimized for item diversity (Model 2), and one based on IRT (Model 3). We hypothesized (**H2**) that the IRT model would be superior to the other two models.

The third aim was to evaluate the convergent, concurrent, and incremental evidence for the validity of the NMAS-BF using latent variables. The use of latent instead of manifest variables to assess validity is important because prior research has found that many significant correlations calculated from raw scores were not significant when using latent variables (Levant et al., 2016, 2017). Convergent evidence for validity was assessed by examining the correlations between the latent variables of Normative Male Alexithymia (using the NMAS) and alexithymia (using the TAS-20). These two constructs overlap in terms of difficulties in identifying and describing feelings, but do not overlap on the more severe aspects of alexithymia (i.e., externally oriented thinking) on the one hand, nor on the socialized process of restricting the expression of vulnerable and caring emotions on the other hand. Structural and hierarchical regression was used to evaluate the concurrent (unique) and incremental evidence for validity, respectively, of the latent factor of the NMAS-BF by examining relationships with alexithymia (TAS-20) and the restrictive emotionality norm of traditional masculinity ideology (RE). If we find that the NMAS-BF explains both unique and incremental variance in RE when the TAS-20 is in the model that would suggest that the NMAS-BF may be tapping a form of alexithymia that is more directly related to men's gender role socialization than the TAS-20.

For this objective the following hypotheses were advanced. **H3**: convergent evidence for validity would be supported by finding a significant, moderate-to-strong, positive correlation between the latent constructs of Normative Male Alexithymia and alexithymia. **H4**: concurrent evidence for validity would be demonstrated by latent NMAS-BF scores uniquely predicting latent restrictive emotionality scores when latent alexithymia scores are included in the model. **H5**: Incremental evidence would be found for validity by NMAS-BF scores significantly predicting variance in restrictive emotionality scores above and beyond that predicted by alexithymia scores.

METHOD

Participants

The present study uses data from a larger project, from which no publications have yet occurred. A total of 505 men were included in the data analysis. Participants ranged in age from 19 to 73 years, with a mean of 35.28 (*SD* = 11.08, median = 33, mode = 26). In regard to race/ethnicity, a majority of participants who responded to this question identified as White (373, 73.9%), and 57 (11.3%) identified as Asian or Asian American, 26 (5.1%) as Black, 24 (4.8%) as multiracial, 16 (3.2%) as Hispanic, 5 (0.8%) as American Indian, and 4 (0.8% of the total sample) did not respond to this question. Regarding sexual orientation identity, most (456, 90.3%) participants reported their sexual orientation as heterosexual, although 21 (4.2%) indicated they were bisexual, 18 (3.6%) indicated they were gay, and 5 (1.0%) indicated a different identity. Five participants (1.0%) did not respond to this question.

Recruitment and Survey Procedures

The study was approved by the University IRB. Community-dwelling participants were recruited using Amazon's Mechanical Turk (MTurk) service. Data obtained from MTurk has been demonstrated to be valid and reliable when appropriate selection criteria and attention checks are used (Casler et al., 2013; Peer et al., 2014), as was the case in this study. All participants were provided with a link to a Qualtrics website, which hosted the study. After completing the informed consent page, participants filled out the questionnaires and were provided with an educational debriefing. The survey contained two validity check items (e.g., "Please check strongly agree"; 30 participants were removed from the data set for failing to correctly respond to the validity check item and are not included in any analyses. Following completion of the study, credit was granted through an automated link between the Qualtrics survey and MTurk.

Sample Size Considerations

For the exploratory factor analysis, we used the MacCallum et al. (1996, Table 6.4) criteria. With 20 observed variables, there were 210 degrees of freedom, indicating that the minimum N is < 178. We had randomly selected 247 cases from the full data set of 505, which is more than adequate. For the CFA, we used the remaining 258 cases, and for the validity analyses we used the full data set of 505. Kline (2016) recommended a minimum of ten participants for every freely estimated parameter. The CFAs had 18 parameters, requiring 180 participants. Our N of 258 exceeds this number. The validity analysis using structural regression had 36 parameters, requiring 360 participants. Our N of 505 exceeds this number.

Measures

Demographic Questionnaire. This questionnaire inquired about gender, age, race/ethnicity, and sexual orientation.

Normative Male Alexithymia Scale (NMAS). The NMAS (Levant et al., 2006) is a 20-item inventory designed to assess Normative Male Alexithymia. Participants answered questions about their own experience of emotions on a seven-point scale (1 = *strongly disagree*; 7 = *strongly agree*), with higher scores indicating greater Normative Male Alexithymia. A sample item is "It is difficult for me to reveal my innermost feelings, even to close friends." Seven items are reverse-scored. NMAS scores were derived by taking a mean of the individual item scores, after recoding the reverse-scored items. The scale was constructed using two samples of mostly White university students (sample 1 = 248 men; sample 2 = 407 men and women). Exploratory and confirmatory factor analyses indicated that the NMAS consisted of a single 20-item factor. As discussed above, scores on the NMAS displayed evidence of internal consistency, test-retest reliability, and validity, but did not have adequate fit statistics in the CFA.

Toronto Alexithymia Scale (TAS-20). The TAS-20 (Bagby et al., 1994) is the most widely used measure of alexithymia, a construct referring to a cluster of characteristics including difficulty identifying and describing feelings, and externally oriented thinking. Participants rated their agreement with 20 statements on a five-point scale (1 = *strongly disagree*; 5 = *strongly agree*), with higher scores indicating greater alexithymia. A sample item is "I am often confused about what emotion I am feeling." Five items are reverse-scored. TAS-20 total scores were derived by taking a mean of the individual item scores after recoding the reverse-scored items. The TAS-20 was developed using a derivation sample of 965 university students, both men and women, to conduct an EFA, and was confirmed with two samples of men and women: 401 university students, and 218 psychiatric outpatients. The scale developers reported total scale coefficient α's from .80 to .83 in the three different samples. Convergent evidence for validity has been demonstrated by negative associations with closely related constructs such as psychological mindedness, need-for-cognition, affective orientation, and emotional intelligence (see Taylor, 2004, for a summary of research using a broad array of student, community, and clinical samples).

Restrictive Emotionality (RE) subscale of the Male Role Norms Inventory-Short Form. RE is one of seven three-item subscales of the MRNI-SF (Levant et al., 2013), which measures the endorsement of traditional masculinity ideology. The scale was developed using data from 1017 university men and women, who were mostly White and heterosexual. It was subsequently used in two samples diverse in terms of race/ethnicity and sexual orientation: Levant et al., 2015; McDermott et al., 2017). Participants responded on a seven-point scale (1 = *strongly disagree*; 7 = *strongly agree*). RE scores are derived by taking a mean of the individual item scores, with higher scores indicating greater endorsement of the restrictive emotionality norm. A sample item is: "Men should be detached in emotionally charged situations." No items are reverse-scored. Levant et al. (2016) reported an alpha coefficient of .82. Using structural equation modeling (SEM), RE showed significant correlations with a latent NMAS factor, the Conformity to Masculine Norms Inventory-46 Emotional Control specific factor, and Gender Role Conflict Scale-SF Restrictive Emotionality first-order factor, providing concurrent evidence for validity (Levant et al., 2016).

Data Analytic Procedures

Overview. Exploratory factor analysis of the 20 NMAS items was conducted using Principle Axis Factoring to assess the dimensionality of the scale. We then generated the three candidate models of the NMAS-BF as defined above. We planned *a priori* to generate six item versions of the NMAS-BF to accomplish two goals. First, we used a multiple of three because construction of latent variables in SEM requires use of at least three manifest variables to indicate a latent factor without causing local identification problems (Little et al., 2002). Use of a model with a number of items that is a multiple of three also allows for easy construction of balanced item parcels and would be useful to future applications of the NMAS-BF. Second, we intended for the NMAS-BF to be a brief scale because the construct assessed would likely be only one of several assessment instruments included in future studies, and brevity would minimize participant burden. Finally, the candidate models of the NMAS-BF were compared in a separate sample using CFA.

Statistical analyses. The exploratory factor analyses, descriptive statistics, and multiple regressions were calculated using SPSS 25. The IRT analysis was conducted using Winsteps version 3.92 (Linacre, 2016). For the CFAs and testing of hypotheses **H2** through **H4**, M*plus* v.8 (Muthén & Muthén, 1998–2017) was used. The overall fit of all CFA models was assessed with the scaled chi-square goodness-of-fit test. However, because this statistic is dependent on sample size, it is overly sensitive to trivial sources of model misfit when sample sizes are large, as in the current study (Cheung & Rensvold, 2002). Thus, a set of alternative fit indices was consulted to determine whether a model demonstrates adequate fit (Kahn, 2006). These indices and the criteria used to assess their values (see Kline, 2016) were the: (a) Comparative Fit Index (CFI) and (b) Tucker–Lewis Index (TLI), which for both indices values of > .90 indicate reasonable fit, and values of > .95 indicate good fit; (c) Root Mean Square Error of Approximation (RMSEA), where good model fit is suggested by values of .05 or lower and values between .05 and .08 suggest reasonable fit; and (d) Standardized Root Mean Square Residual (SRMR), for which values of .05 or lower indicate good model fit, and values of less than .10 are considered acceptable.

For the concurrent validity hypothesis (H3) the recommendations of Russell et al. (1998) and Kline (2016) were followed, and three to four item parcels were created from the manifest variables for the Toronto Alexithymia Scale-20 and the NMAS-BF, the only instruments that had six or more observed items. Item parcels were created by performing principle axis exploratory factor analyses with one-factor solutions for the items comprising this scale. Iterative assignment of items into each one of the parcels was done to ensure that parcel loadings were balanced (Russell et al., 1998). For the three-item Restrictive Emotionality subscale of the MRNI-SF, the observed items were used to assess the latent factors.

RESULTS

Preliminary Analyses

Missing data, outliers, and normality. Thirty participants were removed from the data set for failing to correctly respond to the validity check item. Among the remaining participants, a low level of missing data was observed at the item level (0.2% to 0.6% missing responses per item). The average percentage of missing responses per participant over all items was less than 1%, which is below Parent's (2011) cut-off of 10% for using available item analysis. In addition, there were no other major complicating concerns (e.g., low sample size, poor internal reliability of scales). Thus, we proceeded to analyze the data as recommended by Parent (2011), following the simplest path: no missing values were imputed; rather, all available responses for each item were used in the analysis.

The three scales (NMAS, TAS-20, and RE) evidenced no univariate outliers (i.e., z-scores > 3.29). Likewise, the same scales yielded eight multivariate outliers (1.58% of the sample) as evidenced by Mahalanobis distance procedures. Given the relatively small percentage of outliers and the fact that no outliers were extreme in magnitude, we followed recommendations from Myers et al. (2013) and did not delete or modify outlier cases. The data were only mildly non-normally distributed, with values of skew ranging from –0.42 to 1.28 and values of kurtosis ranging from –1.08 to 0.61.

Exploratory Factor Analyses of Responses to the NMAS

Prior to conducting the exploratory factor analyses, the suitability of the data for factor analysis was assessed. The Kaiser–Meyer–Olkin value was .93, which exceeds the suggested value of .60 (Kaiser, 1974). Bartlett's Test of Sphericity (Bartlett, 1954) was statistically significant, again further supporting the factorability of the correlation matrix. First, Kahn's (2006) recommendation to use parallel analysis (c.f. Hayton et al., 2004) was followed. The analysis indicated that a two-factor structure best represented the dimensionality of the data. To determine which items loaded on the factors, we set the minimum allowable loading at .35 (Tabachnick & Fidell, 2007). Five items that loaded on the second factor did not meet this criterion, which resulted in their removal. We followed Tabachnick and Fidell's (2007) criteria on cross-loading: that items that load .32 or greater on a second factor should be removed, which resulted in the removal of the remaining five items on the second factor, and thus of the second factor. Second, Kaiser's criterion that factors with Eigen values greater than 1 should be retained was followed, which resulted in a four factor solution, from which ten items on the second, third and fourth factors were deleted because of cross-loading with the first factor, resulting in the loss of the those factors. Finally, based on prior research (Levant et al., 2006) and the scree plot[2], the data were analyzed for a one-factor solution, in which the resulting factor loadings ranged from .40 to .85. Thus a one-factor solution was used to create the three candidate models, as shown in Table 6.1. Hypothesis **H1** had specified one-factor dimensionality and thus was supported.

CFA Comparisons of Candidate Models of the NMAS-BF

The basic CFA model tested was a unidimensional model fit to the second data set of 258 participants, in which responses to the six-item NMAS-BF were used as indicators of the hypothesized latent factor. The purpose was to compare the fits of the three candidate models. The results are shown in Table 6.1 (below). Model 1, based on CTT, consisted of the six highest-loading items, whose factor loadings ranged from .74 to .85. The chi-square goodness-of-fit statistic was statistically significant, χ^2 (9) = 92.34; $p < .001$, indicating some sources of misfit. Thus the remaining indices were consulted, and while SRMR was within the guidelines for good fit and CFI was within the guidelines for reasonable fit, TLI and RMSEA were not, indicating marginal to poor fit: CFI = .915; TLI = .858; RMSEA = .192 (90% CI = .157, .228); SRMR = .041. Model 2 was based on a combination of item loading and content, and three high loading items that overlapped with the content of other items were replaced by the next higher loading items. Deleted item 9 overlapped with retained item 14, both referencing innermost feelings; deleted item 20 referenced expressing feelings overlapping with all of the items in the CTT model, so it was replaced with an item tapping difficulty describing feelings (6R); and retained item 15 tapped the sexuality question more directly than deleted item 13. The chi-square goodness-of-fit statistic was also statistically significant, χ^2 (9) = 87.60; $p < .001$, indicating that the null hypothesis of perfect fit should be rejected. Thus, the remaining indices were consulted, and while SRMR was within the guidelines for good fit and CFI was within the guidelines for reasonable fit, TLI and RMSEA were not, indicating marginal to poor fit: CFI = .908; TLI = .847; RMSEA = .186 (90% CI = .152, .223); SRMR = .049.

Finally, Model 3 was based on IRT. All 20 items were entered into the IRT analysis in Winsteps. First, we examined infit and outfit values. Infit and outfit values under .60 or over 1.40 indicate that the patterns of responses were unexpected (i.e., response patterns appear to be influenced by factors other than the construct underlying the measure (Mallinckrodt et al., 2016). Two items were removed from consideration because responses violated accepted infit/outfit criteria. Second, we assessed item difficulty. For scale responses, difficulty reflects whether an item tends to be endorsed or not (i.e., "easy" items are endorsed by more people while "difficult" items are endorsed by fewer). Items were selected for inclusion by dispersing them based on their difficulty scores

TABLE 6.1 Factor Loadings for the Initial EFA

Item		Factor Loading	Model 1	Model 2	Model 3
14.	I have difficulty expressing my innermost feelings.	.85	x	x	
20.	I don't like to talk with others about my feelings.	.84	x		x
9.	It is difficult for me to reveal my innermost feelings, even to close friends.	.76	x		x
13.	I have difficulty expressing my emotional needs to my romantic partner, spouse, or best friend.	.76	x	x	
17.	It is too risky to express my emotions to other people.	.75	x	x	
16.	I do not like to show my emotions to other people.	.74	x	x	
2R.	I feel comfortable expressing my affection to family members and friends.	.55			x
12.	I have difficulty telling others that I care about them.	.69			x
7R.	When someone close to me hurts my feelings, I am able to tell them that I am hurt.	.50			x
10.	If someone asks how I am feeling, I typically say what I am not feeling (e.g., "not too bad").	.40			x
15.	Talking about my feelings during sexual relations is difficult for me.	.70		x	
6R.	I have no trouble putting my feelings into words and discussing them with others.	.63		x	
8R.	I enjoy discussing my innermost feelings with my romantic partner, spouse, or best friend.	.62			
11.	I don't see much value in talking about feelings.	.60			
3.	It does not usually occur to me to deal with my stress by talking about what is bothering me.	.58			
1.	If I am upset or worried I don't like to show it for fear that I will be seen as weak.	.56			
5R.	When asked, I can easily give an account of what I am feeling.	.56			
19R.	I like my feelings.	.52			
18R.	I am comfortable telling someone that I am afraid of something.	.44			
4.	I find it is very hard to cry.	.40			

Note. Model 1 is the model obtained via selection of the highest-loading items from the EFA. Model 2 is the model obtained by using EFA factor loadings and reducing redundancy. Model 3 is the model obtained using IRT to guide item selection.

TABLE 6.2 IRT results

Item number	Difficulty	Infit	Outfit	Excluded	Retained for IRT item set
2	0.41	1.17	1.22		x
19	0.30	1.04	1.14		
5	0.29	0.94	0.91		
11	0.28	1.21	1.19		
12	0.19	0.95	0.95		x
13	0.16	0.83	0.82		
8	0.13	1.08	1.04		
6	0.10	0.91	0.89		
7	0.05	1.08	1.13		x
14	−0.02	0.55	0.57	x	
18	−0.04	1.12	1.19		
15	−0.04	1.02	1.06		
17	−0.08	0.79	0.78		
3	−0.10	1.20	1.40		
9	−0.12	0.77	0.78		x
4	−0.14	1.68	1.87	x	
1	−0.20	1.15	1.19		
20	−0.31	0.60	0.61		x
16	−0.37	0.69	0.68		
10	−0.51	1.39	1.40		x

Note. Excluded items were not included for consideration in the IRT based on elevated infit and/or outfit statistics. Retained items, marked with an "x," were distributed approximately evenly across difficulty values, consistent with IRT procedure. Item numbers in this table correspond to item numbers in Table 6.2.

so as to capture a range of assessments of the construct of NMA. The items selected, along with threshold values, are presented in Table 6.2 (above). No items selected to compose the NMAS-BF demonstrated disordered thresholds. For Model 3, the chi-square goodness-of-fit statistic was statistically significant at only the .05 level, $\chi2$ (9) = 18.05; p = .035. Most of the remaining indices were within the guidelines for good fit or (in the case of RMSEA) reasonable fit, indicating decent fit: CFI = .978; TLI = .963; RMSEA = .063 (90% CI = .016, .105); SRMR = .030. We also determined the test information functions for the three competing models. Test information functions are summaries of item information functions, which are curves that indicate the sensitivity of an item across the range of values on the underlying construct. In the case of the NMAS-BF, which is defined as a unidimensional assessment, the ideal test information function would have broad sides, a high peak, and a smooth bell shape to indicate broad assessment of the underlying construct, maximum contributions of the items to identifying the underlying construct and uniformity in item difficulty, respectively. In addition to the superior fit indices, the IRT model demonstrated a superior test information function curve as the test information function was higher and smoother (Mallinckrodt et al., 2016) (Figure 2). Hence Model 3 was the preferred model, and Hypothesis **H2** was supported. (Figure 6.1)

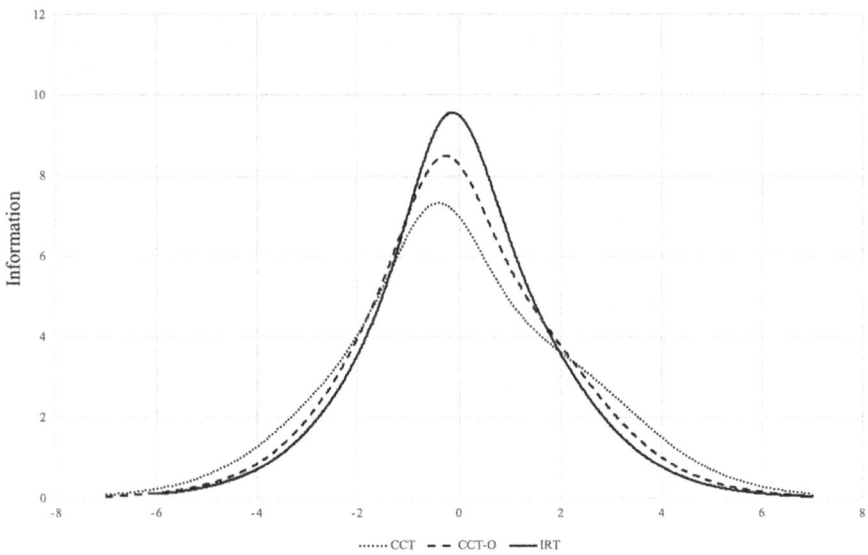

FIGURE 6.1 Test Information Curves for the NMAS-BF

Descriptive statistics. Raw-score-based correlation coefficients, alpha coefficients, means, and standard deviations for the NMAS-BF, TAS-20, and RE scales are presented in Table 6.4. The Cronbach's alpha reliability coefficient for the NMAS-BF was .80, which, according to Ponterotto's and Ruckdeschel's (2007) criteria represents good reliability.

Validity of the NMAS-BF

First, convergent evidence for validity was assessed. The correlation between the latent constructs of Normative Male Alexithymia and alexithymia was significant, moderate-to-strong and positive (.57, $p < .001$), providing convergent evidence for validity and supporting hypothesis **H3**. Second, based on the Chen et al. (2006) guidelines, concurrent evidence for the validity of the latent factor of the NMAS-BF was assessed by constructing a structural regression model. The purpose was to assess whether Normative Male Alexithymia (as assessed by the NMAS-BF) accounted for unique variance in the endorsement of the masculine norm of restricted emotionality (as assessed by RE) when alexithymia (as assessed by the TAS-20) was in the model. In this model, latent factors representing the NMAS-BF and the TAS-20, using parcels as discussed above, were regressed on the latent factor of RE (for which we used observed indicators). The CFA of the measurement model produced reasonable fit to the data, $\chi2$ (41) = 152.70, $p < .001$, CFI = .950, TLI = .933, RMSEA = .073 (90% CI =

TABLE 6.3 CFA Standardized Loadings for NMAS-BF Items

Item	CFA			IRT thresholds				
	Loading	SE	Residual	1	2	3	4	5
N2R. I feel comfortable expressing my affection to family members and friends	0.570	0.050	0.675	−1.03	−0.58	−0.12	0.22	0.53
N12. I have difficulty telling others that I care about them	0.705	0.042	0.502	−1.20	−0.74	−0.22	0.07	0.42
N7R. When someone close to me hurts my feelings, I am able to tell them that I am hurt	0.613	0.047	0.624	−0.93	−0.79	−0.40	−0.09	0.53
N9. It is difficult for me to reveal my innermost feelings, even to close friends	0.658	0.044	0.566	−1.64	−0.91	−0.42	−0.11	0.26
N20. I don't like to talk with others about my feelings	0.787	0.036	0.381	−1.94	−1.05	−0.62	−0.22	0.21
N10. If someone asks how I am feeling, I typically say what I am not feeling (e.g., "not too bad")	0.505	0.054	0.745	−1.46	−0.77	−0.55	−0.34	−0.05

Note. All items loaded onto the latent factor at $p < .001$. *SE* = Standard error.

.061, .086), SRMR = .038. All of the parcels had significant loadings on their respective factors; the standardized loadings ranged from .81 to .82 for the NMAS-BF, and .70 to .85 for the TAS-20. In addition, where manifest indicators were used (i.e., for RE), all indicators had significant loadings on their factor and ranged from .73 to .85. Next, latent factors representing the NMAS-BF and the

TABLE 6.4 Raw Score Scale Intercorrelations, Alpha Coefficients, Means, and Standard Deviations

Scale	2	3	Alpha	Mean	S.D.
1 NMAS-BF	.49**	.28**	.80	4.04	1.32
2 TAS-20	–	.30**	.89	2.39	0.62
3 RE		–	.85	2.60	1.32

Note. NMAS-BF = Normative Male Alexithymia Scale-Brief; TAS-20 = Toronto Alexithymia Scale-20; RE = Restrictive Emotionality Subscale of the Male Role Norms Inventory-Short Form. Scores for the NMAS-BF and RE range from 1 to 7, with higher scores indicating greater Normative Male Alexithymia, and greater endorsement of the masculine norm of restrictive emotionality. Scores for the TAS-20 range from 1 to 5, with higher scores

TABLE 6.5 Structural Regression Paths between the Latent TAS-20 and NMAS-BF Factors and the RE Factor

Path	R^2	Unstandardized	SE	Standardized
Step1: TAS-20	.122***	0.18***	.03	.35***
Step 2: NMAS-BF	.127***	0.31***	.05	.36***

***$p < .001$
(Criterion = RE)

TABLE 6.6 Hierarchical Multiple Regression Analysis of the Regression of TAS-20 and the NMAS-BF on the RE Factor

Predictor	R^2 Change	Unstandardized Coefficients	Standard Errors	Beta Coefficients (Standardized)
Step 1	.088***			
TAS-20		.634***	.091	.297***
Step 2	.025***			
TAS-20		.444***	.103	.189***
NMAS-BF		.212***	.057	.165***

***$p < .001$

TAS-20 were sequentially regressed on the latent factor of RE. This model had exactly the same fit statistics as the measurement model and thus showed reasonable fit to the data. The results are shown in Table 6.5, where it can be seen that the NMAS-BF uniquely predicted restrictive emotionality scores when alexithymia scores were included in the model, supporting hypothesis **H4**. Finally, incremental evidence for validity was examined using hierarchical multiple regression. The results are shown in Table 6.6, where it can be seen that NMAS-BF scores significantly predicted variance in restrictive emotionality scores above and beyond that predicted by alexithymia scores, supporting hypothesis **H5**.

DISCUSSION

The purpose of this study was to develop and assess the psychometric properties of the NMAS-BF. Exploratory factor analysis was used to generate three candidate six-item unidimensional models, which were compared through confirmatory factor analysis. The model based on IRT was superior to models based on CTT and CTT optimized to reduce redundancy. The results also provided evidence for internal consistency reliability, and for convergent, concurrent, and incremental evidence for validity, supporting the use of the NMAS-BF. Future research should further assess the NMAS-BF for test retest reliability and measurement invariance across age, race/ethnicity, and sexual orientation.

There are also implications of the measurement development undertaken in this study for practitioners. The NMAS-BF may be of use to counseling practitioners who wish to quickly assess their clients' ability to express their emotions. Elevated scores on the NMAS-BF may speak to the need to address emotional expression through skill-building while developing client awareness of the benefits and utility of the ability to access and express emotions in terms of interpersonal relationships (Brackett et al., 2011). Also, men may have experienced direct punishment for expressing some emotions during childhood and adolescence and may benefit from explorations of negative learning experiences related to emotional expression (Levant, 2001). There may be cases where discussing a client's overall scores and/or responses to specific items may be of value in the counseling process.

Our use of IRT to inform item selection for the NMAS-BF demonstrates the utility of this approach to item selection. The items selected through IRT encompass a wider range of aspects of Normative Male Alexithymia compared to those selected via CTT, making the NMAS-BF more useful as a brief assessment. Another strength of this study was assessing validity in a latent variable context. The hazards of relying on raw scores have been strikingly demonstrated in other research, where as many as half of the significant correlations using raw scores were not significant using latent variables (Levant et al., 2016, 2017).

There are some limitations of the current study that should be acknowledged. First, the self-report nature of the surveys introduces the possibility of socially desirable responding (SDR). SDR was not measured in our study; however, a recent article demonstrated that SDR is not always a problem (Tracey, 2016). Future investigations using the NMAS-BF are encouraged to continue to address these issues. Second, our sample was composed of mostly White heterosexual men from the United States. Explorations of the construct of Normative Male Alexithymia within more diverse samples and contexts may be useful to inform interventions and clinical work with diverse samples of men. Third, we did not collect data on participants' SES and educational attainment. Future research should collect and report these data. Fourth, participants without internet access were implicitly excluded by the use of MTurk recruitment. Fifth, our evaluation of evidence for validity was limited to just two criterion variables. Future research should expand this to include more of the nomological network.

The NMAS-BF is intended to measure a mild-to-moderate form of alexithymia theorized to be elevated for men due to gender-linked socialization practices – NMA. This theoretical formulation is supported by research demonstrating that the requirement to restrict emotional expression is a central aspect of traditional masculine norms, and that boys are socialized to restrict the expression of vulnerable and caring emotions, we use the word normative to reflect the influence of masculine norms. Although prior research discussed above has found that men experience alexithymia more frequently than do women, that NMAS scores are correlated with the endorsement of traditional masculinity ideology (a construct theorized to be related to masculine socialization), and that in the present study the NMAS-BF demonstrates incremental validity beyond that provided by a current measure of clinical alexithymia (e.g., the TAS) in predicting endorsement of the traditional masculine norm of restrictive emotionality, we have not demonstrated that these differences are due to socialization, and thus we have not yet tested a central element of the GRSP theory. We thus do not know for certain whether NMA (as measured by the NMAS-BF) is related to masculine socialization. In order to definitively say that NMA is related to masculine socialization, we would have to use a measure of masculine socialization, which currently does not exist. Hence, at this stage of instrument development this question cannot be fully answered.

Finally, the present data focused on a singular assessment of the construct of alexithymia; other approaches, such as multi-trait multi-method designs, may be useful in further exploring the nature and implications of Normative Male Alexithymia.

Conclusions

Two main conclusions can be drawn from this study. First, there is evidence supporting the unidimensionality and internal consistency reliability of the NMAS-BF; in addition, there is convergent, concurrent, and incremental evidence for the validity of the NMAS-BF, although additional research is called for in investigating the test-retest reliability and measurement invariance across groups of men defined by race, age, and sexual orientation. Second, the present study demonstrates the advantages of SEM and IRT for assessing the psychometric properties of any scale used in counseling psychology research – in particular for the selection of items, the assessment of dimensionality and the use of latent variables for evaluating evidence for validity.

NOTES

1. Chapter 6, entire chapter. Copyright © 2022 by the American Psychological Association. Reproduced and adapted with permission. The official citation that should be used in referencing this material is Levant, R. F., & Parent, M. C. (2019). The development and evaluation of a brief form of the Normative Male Alexithymia Scale (NMAS-BF). *Journal of Counseling Psychology, 66,* 224–230. http://dx.doi.org/10.1037/cou0000312 No further reproduction or distribution is permitted without written permission from the American Psychological Association.
2. The Eigen value of the first factor was 8.64, accounting for 43.2% of the variance. For comparison's sake, the Eigen value of the second factor was 1.90.

REFERENCES

Bagby, R. M., Parker, J. D. A., & Taylor, G. J. (1994). The twenty-item Toronto Alexithymia Scale—I. Item selection and cross-validation of the factor structure. *Journal of Psychosomatic Research, 38,* 23–32. https://doi.org/10.1016/0022-3999(94)90005-1

Bartlett, M. S. (1954). A note on the multiplying factors for various chi square approximations. *Journal of the Royal Statistical Society, 16* (series B), 296–298. https://doi.org/10.1111/j.2517-6161.1954.tb00174.x

Brackett, M. A., Rivers, S. E., & Salovey, P. (2011). Emotional intelligence: Implications for personal, social, academic, and workplace success. *Social and Personality Psychology Compass, 5,* 88–103. https://doi.org/10.1111/j.1751-9004.2010.00334.x

Casler, K., Bickel, L., & Hackett, E. (2013). Separate but equal? A comparison of participants and data gathered via Amazon's MTurk, social media, and face-to-face behavioral testing. *Computers in Human Behavior, 29,* 2156–2160. https://doi.org/10.1016/j.chb.2013.05.009

Chen, F. F., West, S. G., & Sousa, K. H. (2006). A comparison of bifactor and second-order models of quality of life. *Multivariate Behavioral Research, 41,* 189–225. https://doi.org/10.1207/s15327906mbr4102_5

Cheung, G. W., & Rensvold, R. B. (2002). Evaluating goodness-of-fit indexes for testing measurement invariance. *Structural Equation Modeling, 9,* 233–255. https://doi.org/10.1207/S15328007SEM0902_5

DeVellis, R. F. (2016). *Scale development: Theory and applications.* London: SAGE Publications.

Gignac, G. E., Palmer, B. R., & Stough, C. (2007). A confirmatory factor analytic investigation of the TAS-20: Corroboration of a five-factor model and suggestions for improvement. *Journal of Personality Assessment, 89,* 247–257. https://doi.org/10.1080/00223890701629730

Hayton, J. C., Allen, D. G., & Scarpello, V. (2004). Factor retention decisions in exploratory factor analysis: A tutorial on parallel analysis. *Organizational Research Methods, 7,* 191–205. https://doi.org/10.1177/1094428104263675

Kahn, J. H. (2006). Factor analysis in counseling psychology research, training, and practice: Principles, advances, and applications. *The Counseling Psychologist, 34,* 684–718. https://doi.org/10.1177/0011000006286347

Kaiser, H. H. (1974). An index of factorial simplicity. *Psychometrica, 39,* 31–36. https://doi.org/10.1007/BF02291575

Kline, R. B. (2016). *Principles and practice of structural equation modeling* (4th ed.). New York: Guilford.

Levant, R. F. (2001). Desperately seeking language: Understanding, assessing and treating normative male alexithymia. In G. R. Brooks & G. Good (Eds.), *The new handbook of counseling and psychotherapy for men* (Vol. 1, pp. 424–443). San Francisco: Jossey-Bass.

Levant, R. F., Alto, K. M., McKelvey, D. K., Richmond, K., & McDermott, R. C. (2017). Variance composition, measurement invariance by gender, and validity of the femininity ideology scale-short form. *Journal of Counseling Psychology, 64,* 708–723. https://doi.org/10.1037/cou0000230

Levant, R. F., Good, G. E., Cook, S., O'Neil, J., Smalley, K. B., Owen, K. A., & Richmond, K. (2006). Validation of the normative male alexithymia scale: Measurement of a gender-linked syndrome. *Psychology of Men and Masculinity, 7,* 212–224. https://doi.org/10.1037/1524-9220.7.4.212

Levant, R. F., Hall, R. J., & Rankin. T. J. (2013). Male Role Norms Inventory-Short Form (MRNI-SF): Development, confirmatory factor analytic investigation of structure, and measurement invariance across gender. *Journal of Counseling Psychology, 60,* 228–238. https://doi.org/10.1037/a0031545

Levant, R. F., Hall, R. J., Weigold, I., & McCurdy, E. R. (2016). Construct validity evidence for the male role norms inventory-short form: A structural equation modeling approach using the bifactor model. *Journal of Counseling Psychology, 63,* 534–542. https://doi.org/10.1037/cou0000171

Levant, R. F., & Wong, Y. J. (2013). Race and gender as moderators of the relationship between the endorsement of traditional masculinity ideology and alexithymia: An intersectional perspective. *Psychology of Men and Masculinity, 14,* 329–333. https://doi.org/10.1037/a0029551

Levant, R. F., Wong, Y. J., Karakis, E. N., & Welch, M. W. (2015). Moderated mediation of the relationship between the endorsement of restrictive emotionality and alexithymia. *Psychology of Men and Masculinity, 16,* 459–467. https://doi.org/10.3758/s13428-013-0434-y

Levant, R. F., & Parent, M. C. (2019). The development and evaluation of a brief form of the Normative Male Alexithymia Scale (NMAS-BF). *Journal of Counseling Psychology, 66*(2), 224–233. https://doi-org.ezproxy.uakron.edu:2443/10.1037/cou0000312

Linacre, J. M. (2016). *Winsteps® (Version 3.92.0).* Beaverton, OR: Winsteps.com. Retrieved from http://www.winsteps.com/

Little, T. D., Cunningham, W. A., Shahar, G., & Widaman, K. F. (2002). To parcel or not to parcel: Exploring the question, weighing the merits. *Structural Equation Modeling, 9,* 151–173. https://doi.org/10.1207/S15328007SEM0902_1

MacCallum, R. C., Browne, M. W., & Sugawara, H. M. (1996). Power analysis and determination of sample size for covariance structure modeling. *Psychological Methods*, *1*, 130–149. https://doi.org/1082-989X/96/$3.lXl

Mahalik, J. R., Locke, B. D., Ludlow, L. H., Diemer, M. A., Scott, R. J., Gottfried, M., & Freitas, G. (2003). Development of the conformity to masculine norms inventory. *Psychology of Men & Masculinity, 4*, 3–25. https://doi.org/10.1037/1524-9220.4.1.3

Mallinckrodt, B., Miles, J. R., & Recabarren, D. A. (2016). Using focus groups and rasch item response theory to improve instrument development. *The Counseling Psychologist*, *44*, 146–194. https://doi.org/10.1177/0011000015596437

McDermott, R. C., Levant, R. F., Hammer, J., Hall, R., McKelvey, D., & Jones, Z. (2017). Further examination of the factor structure of the Male Role Norms Inventory-Short Form (MRNI-SF): Measurement considerations for women, men of color, and gay men. *Journal of Counseling Psychology*, *64*, 724–738. https://doi.org/10.1037/cou0000225

Muthén, L. K., & Muthén, B. O. (1998–2015). *Mplus user's guide* (7th ed.). Los Angeles: Muthén & Muthén.

Myers, L. S., Gamst, G., & Guarino, A. J. (2013). *Applied multivariate research: Design and interpretation* (2nd ed.). Thousand Oaks, CA: Sage.

O'Neil, J. M. (2008). Summarizing 25 years of research on men's gender role conflict using the gender role conflict scale. *The Counseling Psychologist, 36*, 358–445. https://doi.org/10.1177/0011000008317057

Parent, M. C. (2011). Handling item-level missing data: simpler is just as good. *The Counseling Psychologist*, *41,* 568–600. https://doi.org/10.1177/0011000012445176

Peer, E., Vosgerau, J., & Acquisti, A. (2014). Reputation as a sufficient condition for data quality on Amazon mechanical turk. *Behavior Research Methods, 46*, 1023–1031. https://doi.org/10.3758/s13428-013-0434-y

Ponterotto, J. G., & Ruckdeschel, D. E. (2007). An overview of coefficient alpha and a reliability matrix for estimating adequacy of internal consistency coefficients with psychological research measures. *Perceptual & Motor Skills*, *105*, 997–1014. https://doi.org/10.2466/PMS.105.7.997-1014

Russell, D. W., Kahn, J. H., Spoth, R., & Altmaier, E. M. (1998). Analyzing data from experimental studies: A latent variable structural equation modeling approach. *Journal of Counseling Psychology*, *45,* 18–29. https://doi.org/10.1037/0022-0167.45.1.18

Tabachnick, B. G., & Fidell, L. S. (2007). *Using multivariate statistics* (5th ed.). Boston: Pearson.

Taylor, G. J. (2004). Alexithymia: Twenty-five years of theory and research. In I. Nyklicek, L. Temoshok, & A. Vingerhoets (Eds.), *Emotional expression and health: Advances in theory, assessment and clinical applications* (pp. 137–153). New York: Brunner-Routledge.

Tracey, T. J. G. (2016). A note on socially desirable responding. *Journal of Counseling Psychology*, *63*, 224–232. https://doi.org/10.1037/cou0000135

PART II
Conclusion

At the beginning of Part II, we discussed the importance of the scientific process of scale development. Throughout this section, we highlighted three major measures of alexithymia, the TAS-20, NMAS, and NMAS-BF. The TAS-20, which has been in existence for quite some time, was superseded by the NMAS for a particular purpose – that is, it was developed specifically to assess Normative Male Alexithymia for the purpose of assessing emotionally inexpressive men. Seeking a shorter scale using cutting-edge scientific analyses that would measure Normative Male Alexithymia, the NMAS-BF was created and found to be reliable and valid. This process reflected the iterative process of scale development in which old scales are replaced with updated ones and old versions are revised to remain relevant and meet demands for practicality.

Based on the psychometric research reported in this section, the NMAS-BF is the tool of choice that practitioners can use to assess for alexithymia in emotionally inexpressive men. We encourage practitioners to use NMAS-BF scores in the early stages of counseling and psychotherapy to ascertain baseline levels of NMA, and to evaluate the effectiveness of interventions with these clients by looking for improved scores on the NMAS-BF post-intervention.

PART III

Treatment

In this part of the book, we turn our attention to the treatment of emotionally inexpressive men, a phenomenon which we have termed Normative Male Alexithymia.

We first provide manuals for Alexithymia Reduction Treatment (ART). For most clinician readers, treatment is often individual therapy. However, some clinicians have found that many men seem to respond well to men's groups. Thus, we have provided manuals for both individual and group therapy formats.

For those readers who may not be familiar with treatment manuals, such manuals have become very prominent in clinical research. The reason is that if one wants to assess the efficacy of a particular treatment approach, one needs to standardize the way that treatment is provided to actual clients, to be sure that one is measuring the same thing across clients. But the advantages of manuals go beyond their utility for research. They provide the clinician with an outline for each session, and a toolbox of exercises that can be done in the sessions. They also empower the client to undertake their growth on their own through homework exercises.

The ART manuals are sequential and graded, based on Levant's conceptualizations. To begin with, men who cannot identify and describe their emotions may not have a vocabulary of emotion words. In groups that Levant led in the 1990s, he would ask the men to provide words for emotions which he would write down on a blackboard. In a group of five or six men, he might get 30 or so words, 20 of which would describe angry emotions: mad, pissed-off, furious, irritated, annoyed, etc. Another eight or nine words described the effects of stress: stressed-out, zapped, burdened, depleted, burned out. And then there might be one bona fide emotion word, like joy. Thus, the first order of business is to help the men develop a vocabulary of words for emotions, particularly for vulnerable emotions such as sadness or fear (i.e., emotions that make us feel vulnerable) as well as for attachment emotions (i.e., like, love, depend). The manuals include in-session and homework exercises to help the clients develop their emotional vocabulary.

Next, Levant proposed that it might be easier to identify emotions in other people than in oneself, so he experimented with his clients, teaching them about the nonverbal expression of emotions, and developing a homework exercise in which the client would work on identifying emotions in other people.

Third, building on these prior steps, he asked his clients to work on identifying their own emotions using a device he called an emotional response log, which will be explained more fully in the manuals.

Unlike treatment manuals for major approaches to psychotherapy, such as Cognitive Behavioral Therapy or Acceptance and Commitment Therapy, the manuals for ART do not take an entire 50-minute session. Thus, ART can be blended with any approach to psychotherapy.

Finally, in keeping with the theme of evidence-based practice, this section also provides a report of a clinical trial of ART, which shows preliminary evidence of efficacy.

CHAPTER SEVEN

Alexithymia Reduction Treatment (ART): A Manual for a Brief Psychoeducational Intervention for Treating Normative Male Alexithymia – Individual Therapy Format

Ronald F. Levant, Christine M. Williams, and Eric W. Hayden

INTAKE

Client's Presenting Concern

Rarely will a man enter therapy complaining of difficulty expressing emotions. Instead, the assessment process conducted during the first session should help the therapist to uncover a pattern of verbal behavior and presenting concerns that is indicative of normative male alexithymia.

Encourage the client to state the problem in his own words; note patterns of vague responses or a general inability to state exactly how a situation bothers him.

If possible, and otherwise not contraindicated, solicit information from the client's intimate partner, particularly regarding the client's difficulty in expressing emotion.[1]

Take note of reports of general relationship problems, stress related to work, substance abuse, referral from outside sources (e.g., Employee Assistance Program, legal system), problems with anger and aggressive behavior,

DOI: 10.4324/9781003378518-11

complaints of physical symptoms (e.g., tension headaches, muscle pain), sexual addictions and compulsive sexual behavior.[2]

These and other problematic issues are likely what the client can articulate is "wrong" when he first comes to therapy. While the client may not be able to talk about them initially, these will likely become the issues that are later dealt with in therapy.

Traditional Assessment

Agency and therapist-specific assessment practices (e.g., intake procedures) are appropriate and encouraged within this framework and will often guide the therapist in uncovering the above information.

Assessment of Alexithymia: The Emotional Spectrum

Levant's theory of Normative Male Alexithymia forms the basis of this intervention and proposes that the standard emotional socialization experience of boys forces the suppression and repression of emotions in early childhood. In particular Levant sees the caring/attachment emotions (e.g., affection, fondness) and the vulnerable emotions (e.g., fear, sadness) as particularly taboo for boys reared in an environment that subscribes to traditional masculinity ideology. The goal of this formal assessment is to determine to what extent the client is aware of specific emotions in various categories – vulnerable, caring and connection, anger and aggression, lust – and able to put them into words. It seeks also to establish the frequency and intensity of the man's emotions as signs of stress that may be experienced. Provided at the end of this session is the Normative Male Alexithymia Scale-Brief Form (NMAS-BF; see Appendix I-I). This may be administered to the client in a paper and pencil format or used to guide a clinical interview done by the therapist. *It is recommended that if choosing to do a clinical interview that the length and depth of the emotional assessment should be tailored to the individual client.* For example, a man who clearly is unaware of basic emotions such as joy will not have much to say about more subtle emotions such as attachment. It may not be best to pursue his deficit at length during the initial interview.

Restatement of the Complaint and Contracting with the Client

The therapist should try to connect the client's complaint to the projected goals and strategy of therapy. Outline a rudimentary treatment plan for the client.

Initiate the psychoeducation process by explaining that difficulty in identifying and expressing emotions is a process that many men struggle with.

Discuss why and how the first part of therapy will center on exercises to gradually strengthen this ability and help the client build skills.

Provide client with informed consent including the limits of confidentiality.[3]

APPENDIX I-I

Normative Male Alexithymia Scale-Brief Form

DIRECTIONS: Please use the scale below to indicate the extent to which you personally agree or disagree with each statement. There are no right or wrong responses.

1	2	3	4	5	6	7
Strongly Disagree	Disagree	Slightly Disagree	Neutral or Undecided	Slightly Agree	Agree	Strongly Agree

1. I don't like to talk with others about my feelings.
2. It is difficult for me to reveal my innermost feelings, even to close friends.
3. I feel comfortable expressing my affection to family members and friends.
4. I have difficulty telling others that I care about them.
5. When someone close to me hurts my feelings, I am able to tell them that I am hurt.
6. If someone asks how I am feeling, I typically say what I am not feeling (e.g., "not too bad").

Scoring Instructions: To obtain the total score (mean item score), reverse the scoring of reverse-scored items, and take the mean. Reverse scored items = 3, 5.

Interpretation of Scores:

Scores can range from low (1) to high (7). The NMAS-BF was not subjected to a clinical assessment to determine cut-off values, as was the TAS-20, so we recommend using the following scheme (using values reported in the validation study) to interpret scores:

Moderately High: Mean plus one standard deviation = 5.36

Very High: Mean plus two standard deviations = 6.68

CITATION: Levant, R. F., & Parent, M. C. (2019). The development and evaluation of a brief form of the Normative Male Alexithymia Scale (NMAS-BF). *Journal of Counseling Psychology, 66*, 224–230. http://dx.doi.org/10.1037/cou0000312

Individual Therapy: First Session

Orienting to Individual Therapy Using This Manual

Working with clients to help them become aware of and identify their emotions can be thought of as a sort of "pre-therapy" intervention to prepare clients to do the work they need to do. The purpose of this manual is to present an intervention that can be incorporated into your current individual therapy structure.

Each module is a psychoeducational "lesson plan" designed to inform clients and stimulate discussion about the phenomenon under discussion and to solicit your client's experiences. This may make up the majority of a session, especially if the client is struggling with issues of masculinity or gender related issues. It may also be a brief segment of any given session as a client addresses other issues.

Additionally, each module ends with a homework assignment that helps clients put the information into practice. You may or may not choose to use the specific forms that we have provided as guides for the homework. However, the homework itself is an essential piece of the program and is the basis of discussion when clients return for the next session.

Inevitably, there will be clients that do not do one or many of the homework assignments. Indeed, the topics that we ask men to discuss here are likely to be unfamiliar and uncomfortable, and it would be surprising not to have a little resistance. However, this need not be viewed as a failure or a sign of a "resistant" client, with all the negative connotations that go with that label. Instead, it can be used as an opportunity for processing the content of sessions and client's reactions in a non-defensive manner in order to enhance their motivation to participate in therapy more fully.

First Session

It is possible, particularly if the intake session was short, that the majority of the first session will be focused on the formation of the therapeutic alliance, information gathering, and an orientation to therapy. As such, the first piece of psychoeducation is particularly short, and might be nicely incorporated toward the end of the session or during a discussion of what to expect in therapy.

Preliminary Psychoeducation

This sets the stage for therapy by providing a framework for clients to understand how this therapy is likely to be helpful with the problems that they are currently experiencing, as well as what to expect. Points to bring up:

- Difficulties identifying and expressing emotions are not uncommon among men.
- Difficulties identifying and expressing emotions are often the basis for other problems that men have, such as relationship issues, difficulty handling stress, or relying on alcohol to relax.

- Many men often do not discuss emotions and may feel that certain emotions are shameful because of how our culture raises boys (e.g., big boys don't cry, men never admit weakness or vulnerability, etc.).
- Emotions are natural for people of any gender identity, and being able to experience and communicate them can lead to better relationships, less stress, a fuller understanding of what you want out of life, and plenty of other positive things.
- Emotional limitations are a problem that can be solved, rather than being accepted as "the way things are."

INDIVIDUAL: SESSION 2

Review Last Session's Homework

Begin by revisiting how male socialization places rigid limits on the emotional repertoire of men; phrases virtually all men can remember from childhood include "big boys don't cry" and, for athletes, "play through your pain."

Discuss with the client what memories he has of similar instances from his childhood.

Developing Vocabulary for Emotions

Words are the medium through which we become aware of, think about, and express our feelings, and an impoverished emotional vocabulary is a common problem for men who suffer from alexithymia. The first stage of therapy aims to expand the client's working lexicon to embrace a fuller spectrum of feelings.

Depending on the client's general level of intellectual sophistication or education, review the physiology behind emotions:

Emotions have four parts:

1. The emotion itself, originating in the limbic system. The limbic system is the primary control center of emotions, hidden deep within the brain; different parts control different emotions such as fear, aggression, hunger, and sex drive.
2. The concomitant autonomic nervous system and endocrinological reactions: Hormonal and neural reactions that stimulate the body, causing changes in heart rate, respiration, sweating, erections.
3. Musculo-skeletal reactions, which involve changes in muscle tension, facial expression, movement, and behavior.
4. Conscious awareness of the emotion.

In some men, only the first three parts occur; they experience emotions and act on them, without being aware of what they are experiencing.

To enter awareness, emotions must be routed through the higher centers of the cerebral cortex, and words are the medium through which this occurs. One can only filter one's emotions through awareness, and consciously decide what to do about them, if one has words to identify them.

Toward a Fuller Emotional Vocabulary

One must first become aware of the words one already uses to begin to build a vocabulary that reflects the full range of human experience. Clients will come to therapy with varying levels of emotional vocabulary and will need different levels of support.

In session: after introducing the idea of building an emotional vocabulary, review the worksheet (see Appendix II-I) with the client. The instructions for the assignment are to "list all the words you can think of to describe emotions." You may choose to start the assignment with the individual in session or have him complete it on his own.[4] Offer a few concrete examples of "emotion words," such as fear and sadness.

Homework assignment: Without using a dictionary or other source, take 20 minutes each, on two separate occasions, this week to list all the emotional words you can think of. Coach the clients to think about emotions they have seen others express (e.g., wives, children, mothers).

APPENDIX II-I

Session II: Homework

List below all the emotion words you can think of. If you get stuck, think about emotions you have seen those around you express. Spend 20 minutes two nights this week trying to think of all that you can.

_____

_____   _____

_____   _____

_____   _____

_____   _____

_____   _____

_____

_____   _____

_____   _____

_____   _____

_____   _____

_____   _____

Appendix II-I Additional Resource

In the following pages, we have provided a rather extensive alphabetical list of emotion words that may be helpful for some clients. This list was reprinted by permission from Rhoda Mills Sommer, LCSW whose website is: https://therapyideas.net/wp content/uploads/2014/04/feelingwordlist.pdf

abandoned	burdened	determined	entertaining	humility
acknowledged	callous	devious	envious	humorous
adequate	calm	different	equal	hungry
affectionate	candid	diligent	euphoric	hurt
afraid	capable	diminished	evil	hysterical
aggressive	captivated	direction	exhausted	idealistic
aggrieved	careful	dirty	expectant	ignorant
agitated	caring	disappointed	failure	ignored
agony	challenged	disbelief	faint	ill
alert	charming	discontent	fair/unfair	impish
alive	cheated	disdainful	fearful	important
alone	cheerful	disembodied	feisty	imposed upon
amazed	childish	disgusted	foolish	impressed
ambitious	clever	dishonored	fragile	impulsive
ambivalent	collapsed	disillusioned	frail	incompetent
amused	combative	disintegrating	free	independent
anger	competitive	disinterested	fresh	inequality
annoyed	condemned	dismayed	friendly	infatuated
anxious	confident	disorientated	frigid	infuriated
apathetic	confused	disrespected	frustrated	innocence
apologetic	conspicuous	dissatisfied	full	insecure
approved of	content	distracted	fun	insightful
arrogant	contrite	distracted	furtive/secretive	insignificant
ashamed	coy	distraught	fury	inspired
assertive	crazy	distressed	generous	intimidated
astounded	creative	distrustful	glad	intolerant
at a loss	creepy	disturbed	glamorous	involved
at ease	cruel	divided	gloomy	irritable
attractive	crummy	dominant	good	irritated
awe/reverence	crushed	down	grateful	isolated
awkward	culpable	drained	great	jealous
backward	curious	driven	greedy	jittery
bad	dead	drowning	grief	joy

balanced
barren
bashful
beautiful
believed
bemused
benevolent
betrayed
bitter
bold
bored
bothered
brave
brilliant
loving/loved
loyalty
lucidity
lucky
lustful
mad
madness/insanity
making amends
malevolence
manipulated
manipulative
marooned
masochistic
mature
mean
mechanical
meek
mindless
miserable
miserly
misery
mixed up
morose
murderous
myopic
mysterious
naïve
nausea
needed
needy
nervous
nervous
nice
nostalgic
not cared for
numb
nutty
obnoxious
obsessed
odd
open
opposed
outraged

deceitful
deceived
decimated
defeated
deliberate
delighted
dependable
dependent
depressed
desirous
despair
desperate
destructive
detached
peaceful
persistent
petrified
phony
picked on
pity/pitiful
placid
playful
pleasant
pleased
pleasure
pointless
polite
positive
powerful
pragmatic
precarious
preoccupied
pressure
pressured
pretty
pride/proud
prim
prissy
profound
protective
proud
punished
pure
pushed out
put down
puzzled
quarrelsome
quick
quiet
rageful
realistic
reasonable
reconciled
refreshed
regretful
rejected
relaxed

dubious
dull
dumb
eager
ecstatic
edgy
elated
electrified
embarrassed
empathy
empty
enchanted
energetic
enjoying
resentful
respect
responsible
restless
reverent
revulsion
rewarded
ridiculous
righteous
rotten
rough
sad
sadistic
safe
sane
sated
satisfied
saturated
scared
screwed up
secure
self sacrifice
selfish
sensitive
sensual
servile
settled
sexy
shallow
sharp
shocked
shrewd
shrewish
shy
significant
silly
skeptical
sleepy
slow
sly/sneaky
small
smart
sneaky

guilty
happy
hated/hateful
healthy
heartsick
helpful
helpless
high & mighty
homesick
honest
honorable
hopeless
horrible
humble
spiritual
startled
sterile
sterile
stingy
stormy
stressed
strong
stuck
stuffed
stupefied
stupid
submerged
submissive
subversive
suffering
suffocated
superior
sure
surprised
surprising
surrendering
suspicious
sympathetic
sympathy
talented
talkative
temporarily
tempted
tenacious
tenderness
tense
tentative
terrible
terrific
terrified
thankful
threatened
thrilled
tight
tired
touchy
tough

jumpy
kind
laughter
lazy
lecherous
left out
let down
lonely
longing
loose
losing
loss
lost
love
triumphant
tyranny
ugly
uncaring
uncomfortable
uneasy
ungrateful
unique
unsettled
upset
vague
vampish
vicious
victimized
violent
vital
vivacious
vulgar
vulnerable
warm
wayward
weak
weepy
well being
whiney
wicked
winsome
wishful
wonderful
wondering
worried
zany

overwhelmed	relieved	solemn	tragic
pain	remorse	sorrowful	tragic
panicked	repulsion	sorry	treacherous

INDIVIDUAL: SESSION 3

Homework Review

Have the client review and share the lists of emotions he came up with. Have the client organize the list into categories and look to fill in holes.

Pay special attention to missing vulnerable (e.g., fear, sadness) or caring (e.g., affection, tenderness) emotions.

Review the notions of traditional male emotion socialization and emotional limitation. It is likely that some clients may not be "buying into" the ideas being presented. Through silence, unsupportive comments, or active challenges they may express these ideas. At the same time, you may find that other clients will spontaneously offer opinions or experiences that support the ideas. It is important to remain open to client challenges and help them work toward an understanding of the concepts and themselves at their own pace.

Learning to Read the Emotions of Others

The twofold importance of this next step should be made clear to the client. The ultimate aim of the program is to develop the ability to become aware of and identify emotions, and it is often easier to start with the emotions of others rather than one's own. Moreover, in and of itself, the ability to relate empathically to the feelings of others immeasurably enriches relationships.

Men and women are equally good at seeing things from another person's perspective, which is the **cognitive foundation for empathy**.

Gender role socialization strengthens **emotional empathy** in women, as they are trained as girls to infer how others feel (i.e., emotional empathy). They do this by vicariously experiencing the other person's feelings. Alexithymic men, who cannot identify and describe their own feelings would be hard pressed to vicariously experience the other person's feelings.

Men develop a different skill. They are trained from their gender role socialization as boys to infer, from their understanding of another person's viewpoint, what that person is going to do, which Levant has termed "**action empathy**."

The goal is to build on the cognitive foundation for empathy and on skills related to action empathy in order to develop emotional empathy.

One good way to determine what a person is feeling is to look for nonverbal cues

Nonverbal Cues

To provide a basic tool for the homework, devote some time to didactic instruction, drawing the client's attention to the following categories of nonverbal cues.

- Facial expression: Most people are aware of the expressions for basic emotions such as fear, anger, and happiness. More nuanced expressions for surprise, shame, and sadness begin to become apparent to the careful observer.
- Tone of voice: Suggest that the timbre, pace, volume, and quality of the voice can convey happiness, fear, anger, or sadness.
- Paralinguistic cues: Sighs, cries, gasps are all indicative of emotions, often strong ones.
- Body language: General posture and movement give a lot of information about the emotions of others. The therapist might point out some basics – how a closed posture, with arms and legs crossed, and an open, relaxed sitting position suggest different feeling states.

Homework Assignment

Ask the client to watch other people, in conversation, on the job, at home, or in social situations, with the conscious intention of identifying their emotions. It is often useful to suggest that the client practice his emotion-reading skills with characters on TV or in movies. Movies from the 1950s and earlier are often particularly helpful; the unfamiliar tone and setting might make it easier to identify the emotions displayed. And the more stylized acting in many older films makes emotions more accessible to the observer.

Ask yourself, "What is he/she feeling?"

Use the vocabulary list developed in Step 1, or the additional resource list of emotions to identify the feeling.

Write down the situation the person is in and what they are likely *feeling*. (Remind clients **not** to fall back on what the person is *doing* or *thinking*. Use feeling words).

Appendix III-I presents a possible format for clients to use.

Some clients may need to spend more than a week on this stage of therapy. Once they have mastered the basics, the practice of emotional empathy will be a recurring focus as the therapy progresses. Being able to read others' emotions will start to occur as clients recount stories in therapy. Of course, the therapist models emotional empathy by providing it to the client throughout the course of therapy. Many clients pick up on this, commenting that the therapist seems to be doing what they themselves are learning to do.

APPENDIX III-I

Emotional Empathy Exercise

Using your list of emotions developed in the first homework, watch the reactions of people around you at home, work, in public, or even on TV or in a movie. Record what the situation is that is occurring, and what it is they are likely *feeling*. Remember, try to guess what they are feeling (e.g., happiness, surprise, concern, disgust), not what they're doing or thinking.

Situation	Emotion(s)

INDIVIDUAL: SESSION 4

Homework Review

Clients should be returning with their experiences of trying to read emotions in others. Some will have made good progress with the assignment, while others may still be having difficulty identifying the emotions of others. Additionally, it is possible that a client may have completed the assignment but have focused on actions or thoughts of the others around them.

Have the client describe the nonverbal cues they picked up on.

Discuss what problems the client had in trying to read the emotions of others, especially for those who felt that they couldn't do it.

Discuss any insights or benefits the client had from being able to read someone else's emotions; were there any benefits they could see happening?

Throughout subsequent sessions, referring back to reading the emotions of others will become part of the natural discussion around situations that the client will present.

Some clients are likely to express resistance to the exercises or the concepts in general. Remember, modeling through empathic understanding or self-disclosure of one's own or other clients' experiences with the techniques may help the client see the value of the work.

Keeping an Emotional Response Log

Applying the emotional vocabulary and emotional empathy skills developed in prior sessions to the more difficult task of reading one's own emotions is the summit of the process. At this point, it is vital to acknowledge the progress that the client has made and give full credit for obstacles overcome.

By now, the clients' motivation is apt to be strengthened by a growing sense of mastery and discovery. They have begun to make connections that make life more interesting and richer. A vision of new possibilities may well draw him into the challenge of turning his attention from the feelings of others to his own.

The essential tool for putting the client's own emotions into words is a formal record, the "emotional response log," which he keeps for the duration of therapy. Each entry will have three parts:

- The feeling, bodily sensation, or sign of stress that he first becomes aware of. (For many men, this will be the undifferentiated "buzz" of emotional arousal.)
- The context – social situation, conversation, event, or circumstance – in which it occurred. Who is doing what to whom and how does it affect him?
- The identified emotion. Suggest that he go through his vocabulary list to figure out the words that best describe the experience that he is having.

Homework

The client will be asked to spend the next week working on their emotional response log. It is important to have a convenient, easily carried format in which to keep the log. A small notebook, index cards, or a Notes file in a phone are possible suggestions. Appendix IV-I presents a possible format for clients to use.

APPENDIX IV-I

Emotional Response Log

Date	Sensation, sign of stress, or feeling	Context/circumstance	Words to describe emotion

INDIVIDUAL: SESSION 5

Review of Homework

The client should also return with their emotional response logs for this week. This task typically takes two or more sessions to master, so this week will review and expand on the material presented in the last session.

Have the client discuss experiences from the week and what emotions they were able to pick out from their experiences.

Look for reliance on the old repertoire of emotions, such as anger and "stress" that are typically recorded during first tries at this assignment.

"Don't accept anger at face value" is a useful instruction. If a client can relinquish the empowering experience of anger, he is likely to find vulnerable emotions like fear and hurt underneath.

Men who repeatedly record being "stressed out" should be encouraged to tease apart their unease in search of more specific feelings.

Continue to work with resistance to the exercises or the concepts in general.

The Experience of Shame

It is in this stage of therapy that shame is most likely to become an obstacle. The therapist must be particularly supportive, making use of the psychoeducational groundwork already established.

- Refer back to the axiom that all emotions are "natural" and "human."
- Resistance will be overcome to the extent that the emotional expansion process can be reframed as courageous rather than weak.
- Praise clients for being willing to "brave the shame" of violating male socialization taboos.

Discuss the difference between *experiencing* and *expressing* emotions. Being able to experience his emotions opens up choices for the client. It does not mean having to show all of his emotions to everyone. In fact, he is now gaining control of his emotional reactions and will be able to choose when and what to express. In short, by identifying and describing his emotions, he is routing them through his neocortex, given him the power to think about them and to choose what he wants to do with them.

Practice

As with any developing skill, practice is the key to making emotional self-awareness automatic and integrating it into the client's day-to-day life. As sessions continue, feedback from the therapist can help clients identify the emotions that they have experienced in situations, or even that they are experiencing in the course of therapy. Raising questions of "How did you feel?" and "How do you think she felt?" will continue to reinforce the client's developing skills.

Homework

The same assignment will be repeated for at least the next session, if not the next few sessions. Reminders of working to get underneath the experiences of anger and stress should direct the client to work to uncover their full range of emotions, especially the vulnerable (e.g., fear, sadness) and caring (e.g., tenderness, affection) ones.

INDIVIDUAL: SESSION 6

Review Homework

- As before, check in with the client to review progress in identifying the emotions of others. Hopefully the client's emotional response log reflects a growing awareness of their emotions.
- Review the log from the past week.
- Ask for instances where the client finds that they've uncovered a new emotional experience or were able to keenly identify previously untapped emotions.
- Help clients, both those who are, or are not, having success, process roadblocks in uncovering emotions.

Readminister the NMAS-BF

- See Appendix V-I.
- Compare the current score to the earlier one and discuss how the score has changed. Look at individual items that were scored differently and discuss.
- Discuss benefits or changes that the client is experiencing from being able to identify their emotions.
- Continue to work with the resistance of the client to the exercises or the concepts in general.

Moving Forward

The client's life itself is likely to provide the most effective positive feedback. These skills are self-reinforcing for most: men feel empowered and energized as they learn them. Clients become highly motivated when they discover that their emerging empathy, openness, and communication skills reduce conflict and increase harmony in their family lives.

Deeper Issues

As the client becomes more emotionally self-aware, he will start to make connections to other problems, and the relevance of other issues are likely to surface. The conversations will turn from understanding and moving beyond a state of Normative Male Alexithymia to conversations about the difficulties in clients' lives. The therapist simply follows this process as it leads into deeper areas and directs the clients' application of their emerging emotional skills to work on them.

APPENDIX VI-I

Normative Male Alexithymia Scale-Brief Form

DIRECTIONS: Please use the scale below to indicate the extent to which you personally agree or disagree with each statement. There are no right or wrong responses.

1	2	3	4	5	6	7
Strongly Disagree	Disagree	Slightly Disagree	Neutral or Undecided	Slightly Agree	Agree	Strongly Agree

1. I don't like to talk with others about my feelings.
2. It is difficult for me to reveal my innermost feelings, even to close friends.
3. I feel comfortable expressing my affection to family members and friends.
4. I have difficulty telling others that I care about them.
5. When someone close to me hurts my feelings, I am able to tell them that I am hurt.
6. If someone asks how I am feeling, I typically say what I am not feeling (e.g., "not too bad").

Scoring Instructions: To obtain the total score (mean item score), reverse the scoring of reverse-scored items, and take the mean. Reverse scored items = 3, 5.

Interpretation of Scores:

Scores can range from low (1) to high (7). The NMAS-BF was not subjected to a clinical assessment to determine cut-off values, as was the TAS-20, so we recommend using the following scheme (using values reported in the validation study) to interpret scores:

Moderately High: Mean plus one standard deviation = 5.36
Very High: Mean plus two standard deviations = 6.68

NOTES

1. It is unusual for a man to come in complaining of difficulty in expressing emotions. Frequently, the visit has been instigated, at least in part, by the client's wife or intimate partner; she typically is the one who has identified his emotional constriction as a problem.
2. Normative Male Alexithymia has been theorized to relate to these clinical syndromes in that they are thought to be the result of maladaptive coping strategies the man has developed in lieu of an ability to verbally process his emotions and seek social support.
3. Include any state statutes regarding the mandatory reporting laws (e.g., child and elder abuse), and limitations of confidentiality based upon the states statutes of duty to protect or duty to warn. Please refer to your state's relevant legal code and all professional ethical guidelines.
4. You might choose to start the homework in session or just send it home depending on your sense of the individual. You want to start the homework with those clients without a fuller lexicon to get them started.

CHAPTER EIGHT

Alexithymia Reduction Treatment (ART): A Manual for a Brief Psychoeducational Intervention for Treating Normative Male Alexithymia – Group Therapy Format

Ronald F. Levant, Christine M. Williams, and Eric W. Hayden

INTAKE[1]

Client's Presenting Concern

Rarely will a man enter therapy complaining of difficulty expressing emotions. Instead, the assessment process conducted during the first session should help the therapist to uncover a pattern of verbal behavior and presenting concerns that is indicative of Normative Male Alexithymia.

Encourage the client to state the problem in his own words; note patterns of vague responses (e.g., "I've been feeling bad," "uncomfortable around certain people/topics," "stressed," "confused," "tired a lot lately") or a general inability to state exactly how a situation bothers him.

If possible, and otherwise not contraindicated, solicit information from the client's intimate partner, particularly regarding the client's difficulty in expressing emotion.[2]

Take note of reports of general relationship problems, stress related to work, substance abuse, referral from outside sources (e.g., Employee Assistance

DOI: 10.4324/9781003378518-12

Program, legal system), problems with anger and aggressive behavior, complaints of physical symptoms (e.g., tension headaches, muscle pain), sexual addictions and compulsive sexual behavior.[3]

These and other problematic issues are likely what the client can articulate is "wrong" when he first comes to therapy. While the client may not be able to talk about them initially, these will likely become the issues that are later dealt with in therapy.

Traditional Assessment

Agency and therapist-specific assessment practices (e.g., intake procedures) are appropriate and encouraged within this framework and will often guide the therapist in uncovering the above information.

Assessment of Alexithymia: The Emotional Spectrum

Levant's theory of Normative Male Alexithymia forms the basis for Alexithymia Reduction Treatment (ART) and proposes that the standard emotional socialization experience of boys forces the suppression and repression of emotions in early childhood. In particular, Levant sees the caring/attachment emotions (e.g., affection, fondness) and the vulnerable emotions (e.g., fear, sadness) as particularly taboo for boys reared in an environment that subscribes to traditional masculinity ideology. The goal of this formal assessment is to determine to what extent the client is aware of specific emotions in various categories – vulnerable, caring and connection, anger and aggression, lust – and able to put them into words. It seeks also to establish the frequency and intensity of the man's emotions as signs of stress that may be experienced. Provided at the end of this session is the Normative Male Alexithymia ScaleBrief Form (NMAS-BF, see Appendix I-G). This may be administered to the client in a paper and pencil format, or used to guide a clinical interview done by the therapist. *It is recommended that if choosing to do a clinical interview that the length and depth of the emotional assessment should be tailored to the individual client.* For example, a man who clearly is unaware of basic emotions such as joy will not have much to say about more subtle emotions such as attachment. It may not be best to pursue his deficit at length during the initial interview.

Restatement of the Complaint and Contracting with the Client

The therapist should try to connect the client's complaint to the projected goals and strategy of therapy. Outline a rudimentary treatment plan for the client.

Discuss the appropriateness and client preferences for the suggested mode of treatment (i.e., group or individual).

Initiate the psychoeducation process by explaining that difficulty in identifying and expressing emotions is a process that many men struggle with.

Discuss why and how the first part of therapy will center on exercises to gradually strengthen this ability and help the client build skills.

Provide client with informed consent including the limits of confidentiality.[4,5]

APPENDIX I-G

Normative Male Alexithymia Scale-Brief Form

DIRECTIONS: Please use the scale below to indicate the extent to which you personally agree or disagree with each statement. There are no right or wrong responses.

1	2	3	4	5	6	7
Strongly Disagree	Disagree	Slightly Disagree	Neutral or Undecided	Slightly Agree	Agree	Strongly Agree

1. I don't like to talk with others about my feelings.
2. It is difficult for me to reveal my innermost feelings, even to close friends.
3. I feel comfortable expressing my affection to family members and friends.
4. I have difficulty telling others that I care about them.
5. When someone close to me hurts my feelings, I am able to tell them that I am hurt.
6. If someone asks how I am feeling, I typically say what I am not feeling (e.g., "not too bad").

Scoring Instructions: To obtain the total score (mean item score), reverse the scoring of reverse-scored items, and take the mean. Reverse-scored items = 3, 5.

Interpretation of Scores:

Scores can range from low (1) to high (7). The NMAS-BF was not subjected to a clinical assessment to determine cut-off values, as was the TAS-20, so we recommend using the following scheme (using values reported in the validation study) to interpret scores:

Moderately High: Mean plus one standard deviation = 5.36

Very High: Mean plus two standard deviations = 6.68

Citation: Levant, R. F., & Parent, M. C. (2019). The development and evaluation of a brief form of the Normative Male Alexithymia Scale (NMAS-BF). *Journal of Counseling Psychology, 66*, 224–230. http://dx.doi.org/10.1037/cou0000312

GROUP: FIRST SESSION

Orienting to Group Therapy Using This Manual

Working with clients to help them become aware of and identify their emotions can be thought of as a sort of "pre-therapy" intervention to prepare group members to do the work they need to do. The purpose of this manual is to present a system that can be incorporated into your current group therapy structure. It is designed to fit into programs that you already have in place or be the foundation on which to build a more comprehensive program.

Each module is a psychoeducational "lesson plan" designed to inform clients and stimulate group discussion about the phenomenon under discussion and to solicit participants' experiences. This may make up the majority of the group process, if the group is meant to be purely psychoeducational and an end in-and-of-itself. It can also be one component of a group that is also meant to be a therapy group.

Additionally, each module ends with a homework assignment that helps participants put the information into practice. You may or may not choose to use the specific forms that we have provided as guides for the homework. However, the homework itself is an essential piece of the program and is the basis of discussion when clients return for the next session. Inevitably, there will be participants that do not do one or many of the homework assignments. Indeed, the topics that we ask men to discuss here are likely to be unfamiliar and uncomfortable, and it would be surprising not to have a little resistance. However, this need not be viewed as a failure or a sign of a "resistant" client, with all the negative connotations that go with that label. Instead, it can be used as an opportunity for processing the content of sessions and client's reactions in a non-defensive manner in order to enhance their motivation to participate more fully.

First Session

It is expected that the majority of the first session will be focused on the formation of the group, introductions, setting out rules and expectations, and other processes related to beginning any sort of group therapy. As such, the first piece of psychoeducation is particularly short, and might be nicely incorporated toward the end of the session or during a discussion of what to expect in therapy.

Preliminary Psychoeducation

This sets the stage for therapy by providing a framework for participants to understand how this therapy is likely to be helpful with the problems that they are currently experiencing, as well as what to expect. Points to bring up:

Difficulties identifying and expressing emotions are not uncommon among men.

Difficulties identifying and expressing emotions are often the basis for other problems that men have, such as relationship issues, difficulty handling stress, or relying on alcohol to relax.

Men often do not discuss emotions and may feel that certain emotions are shameful because of how our culture raises boys (e.g., big boys don't cry, men never admit weakness or vulnerability, etc.).

Emotions are natural for people of any sex or gender identity, and being able to experience and communicate them can lead to better relationships, less stress, a fuller understanding of what you want out of life, and plenty of other positive things.

Emotional limitations are a problem that can be solved, rather than being accepted as "the way things are."

GROUP: SESSION 2

Review Last Session's Discussion

Begin by revisiting how male socialization places rigid limits on the emotional repertoire of men; phrases virtually all men can remember from childhood include "big boys don't cry," "don't be a wuss," and, for athletes, "play through your pain."

Solicit participants to provide examples that continue the discussion from last time.

Developing a Vocabulary for Emotions

Words are the medium through which we become aware of, think about, and express our feelings, and an impoverished emotional vocabulary is a common problem for men who suffer from alexithymia. The first stage of therapy aims to expand the client's working lexicon to embrace a fuller spectrum of feelings.

Depending on the group's general level of intellectual sophistication or education, review the psychophysiology behind emotions.

Emotions have four parts:

- The emotion itself, originating in the limbic system. The limbic system is the primary control center of emotions, hidden deep within the brain; different parts control different emotions such as fear, aggression, hunger, and sexual arousal.

- The concomitant autonomic nervous system and endocrinological reactions: Hormonal and neural reactions that stimulate the body, causing changes in heart rate, respiration, sweating, erections.
- Musculo-skeletal reactions, which involve changes in muscle tension, facial expression, movement, and behavior.
- Conscious awareness of the emotion.

In many men, only the first three parts occur; they experience emotions and act on them, without being aware of what they are experiencing.

To enter awareness, emotions must be routed through the higher centers of the cerebral cortex, and words are the medium through which this occurs. To filter one's emotions through awareness, and consciously decide what to do about them, one must have words to identify them.

Mention that anger is the one emotion that most men are aware of, because it is notably experienced in their musculature and/or acted upon – physically and/or verbally. Facilitate discussion around this by asking men to call out where in their body they notice they carry their anger. This discussion helps set the stage for future sessions in which men are taught to identify more vulnerable emotions by attuning to their bodily reactions.

Toward a Fuller Emotional Vocabulary

One must first become aware of the words one already uses in order to begin to build a vocabulary that reflects the full range of human experience. Clients will come to group therapy with varying levels of emotional vocabulary and will need different levels of support.

In group: After introducing the idea of building an emotional vocabulary, pass around the worksheet (see Appendix II-G). The instructions for the assignment are to "list all the words you can think of to describe emotions." Have the men list as many as they can.[6] Offer a few concrete examples of "emotion words," such as fear and sadness.

Have the men review their lists privately, asking them to look for patterns in their words (e.g., all relate to happiness) or gaps (e.g., no words relate to sadness). Have the men share some of the gaps and patterns that they see. Solicit them to see if anyone listed groups of words related to caring (e.g., affection, tenderness) or vulnerability (e.g., fear, sadness) emotions. Likely, there will be gaps surrounding these emotional words, due to men's socialization experiences.

Homework assignment: Without using a dictionary or other source, take 20 minutes each, on two separate occasions, this week to list all the emotional words you can think of. Coach the participants to think about emotions they have seen others express (e.g., wives, children, mothers).

APPENDIX II-G

In Session Exercise: Session 2

Think about emotions you might feel. Think about emotions that your dating partner, wife, children, sister, or mother might feel. List the ones that come to mind.

APPENDIX II-G

Session II: Homework

List below all the emotion words you can think of. If you get stuck, think about emotions you have seen those around you express. Spend 20 minutes two nights this week trying to think of all that you can.

_____   _____

_____   _____

_____   _____

_____   _____

_____   _____

_____

_____   _____

_____   _____

_____   _____

_____   _____

_____

APPENDIX II-G ADDITIONAL RESOURCE

In the following pages, we have provided a rather extensive alphabetical list of emotion words that may be helpful for some clients. This list was reprinted by permission from Rhoda Mills Sommer, LCSW whose website is: https://therapyideas.net/wp content/uploads/2014/04/feelingwordlist.pdf

abandoned	burdened	determined	entertaining	humility
acknowledged	callous	devious	envious	humorous
adequate	calm	different	equal	hungry
affectionate	candid	diligent	euphoric	hurt
afraid	capable	diminished	evil	hysterical
aggressive	captivated	direction	exhausted	idealistic
aggrieved	careful	dirty	expectant	ignorant
agitated	caring	disappointed	failure	ignored
agony	challenged	disbelief	faint	ill
alert	charming	discontent	fair/unfair	impish
alive	cheated	disdainful	fearful	important
alone	cheerful	disembodied	feisty	imposed upon
amazed	childish	disgusted	foolish	impressed
ambitious	clever	dishonored	fragile	impulsive
ambivalent	collapsed	disillusioned	frail	incompetent
amused	combative	disintegrating	free	independent
anger	competitive	disinterested	fresh	inequality
annoyed	condemned	dismayed	friendly	infatuated
anxious	confident	disorientated	frigid	infuriated
apathetic	confused	disrespected	frustrated	innocence
apologetic	conspicuous	dissatisfied	full	insecure
approved of	content	distracted	fun	insightful
arrogant	contrite	distracted	furtive/secretive	insignificant
ashamed	coy	distraught	fury	inspired
assertive	crazy	distressed	generous	intimidated
astounded	creative	distrustful	glad	intolerant
at a loss	creepy	disturbed	glamorous	involved
at ease	cruel	divided	gloomy	irritable
attractive	crummy	dominant	good	irritated
awe/reverence	crushed	down	grateful	isolated
awkward	culpable	drained	great	jealous
backward	curious	driven	greedy	jittery
bad	dead	drowning	grief	joy
balanced	deceitful	dubious	guilty	jumpy
barren	deceived	dull	happy	kind
bashful	decimated	dumb	hated/hateful	laughter
beautiful	defeated	eager	healthy	lazy
believed	deliberate	ecstatic	heartsick	lecherous
bemused	delighted	edgy	helpful	left out
benevolent	dependable	elated	helpless	let down
betrayed	dependent	electrified	high & mighty	lonely
bitter	depressed	embarrassed	homesick	longing
bold	desirous	empathy	honest	loose
bored	despair	empty	honorable	losing
bothered	desperate	enchanted	hopeless	loss
brave	destructive	energetic	horrible	lost

brilliant	detached	enjoying	humble	love
loving/loved	peaceful	resentful	spiritual	triumphant
loyalty	persistent	respect	startled	tyranny
lucidity	petrified	responsible	sterile	ugly
lucky	phony	restless	sterile	uncaring
lustful	picked on	reverent	stingy	uncomfortable
mad	pity/pitiful	revulsion	stormy	uneasy
madness/insanity	placid	rewarded	stressed	ungrateful
making amends	playful	ridiculous	strong	unique
malevolence	pleasant	righteous	stuck	unsettled
manipulated	pleased	rotten	stuffed	upset
manipulative	pleasure	rough	stupefied	vague
marooned	pointless	sad	stupid	vampish
masochistic	polite	sadistic	submerged	vicious
mature	positive	safe	submissive	victimized
mean	powerful	sane	subversive	violent
mechanical	pragmatic	sated	suffering	vital
meek	precarious	satisfied	suffocated	vivacious
mindless	preoccupied	saturated	superior	vulgar
miserable	pressure	scared	sure	vulnerable
miserly	pressured	screwed up	surprised	warm
misery	pretty	secure	surprising	wayward
mixed up	pride/proud	self sacrifice	surrendering	weak
morose	prim	selfish	suspicious	weepy
murderous	prissy	sensitive	sympathetic	well being
myopic	profound	sensual	sympathy	whiney
mysterious	protective	servile	talented	wicked
naïve	proud	settled	talkative	winsome
nausea	punished	sexy	temporarily	wishful
needed	pure	shallow	tempted	wonderful
needy	pushed out	sharp	tenacious	wondering
nervous	put down	shocked	tenderness	worried
nervous	puzzled	shrewd	tense	zany
nice	quarrelsome	shrewish	tentative	
nostalgic	quick	shy	terrible	
not cared for	quiet	significant	terrific	
numb	rageful	silly	terrified	
nutty	realistic	skeptical	thankful	
obnoxious	reasonable	sleepy	threatened	
obsessed	reconciled	slow	thrilled	
odd	refreshed	sly/sneaky	tight	
open	regretful	small	tired	
opposed	rejected	smart	touchy	
outraged	relaxed	sneaky	tough	
overwhelmed	relieved	solemn	tragic	
pain	remorse	sorrowful	tragic	
panicked	repulsion	sorry	treacherous	

GROUP: SESSION 3

Homework Review

Have participants review and share the lists of emotions that they came up with. If available, use a chalkboard, whiteboard, or something similar to create a list. Have participants help organize lists into categories and look to fill in holes.

Have participants add to their lists and work to categorize the words they came up with as the group discusses the homework.

Pay special attention to missing vulnerable (e.g., fear, sadness) or caring (e.g., affection, tenderness) emotions.

Review the notions of traditional male emotion socialization and emotional limitation.

It is likely that some men may not be "buying into" the ideas being presented. Through silence, unsupportive comments, or active challenges, they may express these ideas. At the same time, you may find that other group members will spontaneously offer opinions or experiences that support the ideas. Some ways to deal with unsupportive comments or active challenges is to ask: "Have others had similar experiences?" or "Does anyone feel differently?" to facilitate discussions.

Several ways to deal with silence is to have members break out into dyads to discuss their reactions to the homework. When members are paired and given directions to discuss something, they likely will talk to each other. The initially lowered threat of talking with only one person often gives members who might otherwise have been silent the confidence to speak in the large group. When the dyad has finished talking, the leader may use some of the following questions to get members to talk in the large group: "What emotions did you and your partner list in common?" "What emotions did you list that were different from your partner?" "What was your reaction to the homework?" "What did the two of you discuss?"

Another way to draw out silent members is to have a round, whereby the leader asks everyone to comment. The comment could come in the form of a phrase or a word. The leaders may instruct the members to comment in any order ("popcorn style") or comment in a clockwise or counter-clockwise ("round robin") fashion if the group is arranged in a circle.

One last option for getting silent members to participate is to have a round in which each person simply rates on a scale of 1 to 10 their "buy in" to the ideas presented so far. Here is an example of how this could be introduced:

> Alright, we've talked a bit about how men are conditioned to hold back expression of certain feelings and how this can cause or make more problems in relationships. So, I'm wondering how much each of you agrees

with all of this. As a way to get a read on this, I'd like to go around the circle and have each of you rate out loud on a scale of 1 to 10 how much you buy into these ideas. A 10 means you agree a lot and a 1 means you think it is a lot of bull.

It may be helpful for the leader to offer members the option to pass on the first go-around in a circle as a way to respect a person's readiness to participate, then come back to him on a second pass.

Learning to Read the Emotions of Others

The twofold importance of this step should be made clear to the group. The ultimate aim of the program is to develop the ability to become aware of and identify emotions, and it is often easier to start with the emotions of others rather than one's own. Moreover, in and of itself, the ability to relate empathically to the feelings of others immeasurably enriches relationships.

On average, people of all gender identities are equally good at seeing things from another person's perspective, which is the **cognitive foundation for empathy**.

Socialization strengthens **emotional empathy** in women, as they are trained to infer how others feel (i.e., emotional empathy).

Men develop a related skill: They are trained to infer what someone else is going to do, which Levant has termed "**action empathy**."

The goal is to build on the cognitive foundation for empathy and on skills related to action empathy in order to develop emotional empathy.

One good way to determine what a person is feeling is to look for nonverbal cues

Nonverbal Cues

To provide a basic tool for the homework, devote some time to didactic instruction, drawing the group's attention to nonverbal cues.

Facial expression: Most people are aware of the expressions for basic emotions such as fear and happiness. More nuanced expressions for surprise, shame, and sadness begin to become apparent to the careful observer.

Tone of voice: Suggest that the timbre, pace, volume, and quality of the voice can convey happiness, fear, anger, or sadness.

Body language: General posture and body movement give a lot of information about the emotions of others. The therapist might point out some basics – how a closed posture, with arms and legs crossed, and an open, relaxed sitting position suggest different feeling states.

Homework Assignment

Watch other people, in conversation, on the job, at home, or in social situations, with the conscious intention of identifying their emotions. It is often useful to suggest that the client practice his emotion-reading skills with characters on TV or in movies. Movies from the 1950s and earlier are often particularly helpful; the unfamiliar tone and setting might make it easier to identify the emotions displayed. And the more stylized acting in many older films makes emotions more accessible to the observer.

Ask yourself, "What is he/she feeling?"

Use the vocabulary list developed in Step 1 to identify the feeling.

Write down the situation the person is in and what they are likely *feeling*. (Remind participants **not** to fall back on what the person is *doing* or *thinking*. Use feeling words).

Appendix III-G presents a possible format for participants to use

Many clients will need to spend more than a week on this stage of therapy. Once they have mastered the basics, the practice of emotional empathy will be a recurring focus as the therapy progresses. Being able to read others' emotions will start to occur as participants recount stories in therapy, or even react to one another. Of course, *the therapist models emotional empathy* by providing it to each client throughout the course of the group. Many clients pick up on this, commenting that the therapist seems to be doing what they themselves are learning to do.

APPENDIX III-G

Emotional Empathy Exercise

Using your list of emotions developed in the first homework, watch the reactions of people around you at home, work, in public, or even on TV or in a movie. Record what the situation is that is occurring, and what it is they are likely *feeling*. Remember, try to guess what they are feeling (e.g., happiness, surprise, concern, disgust), not what they're doing or thinking.

Situation	Emotion(s)

GROUP: SESSION 4

Homework Review

Participants should be returning with their experiences of trying to read emotions in others. Some will have made good progress with the assignment, while others may still be having difficulty identifying the emotions of others. Additionally, it is possible that a client may have completed the assignment but have focused on actions or thoughts of the others around them.

Solicit examples from participants that had success; have the person describe the non-verbal cues they picked up on.

Discuss what problems participants had in trying to read the emotions of others, especially for any who felt that they couldn't do it.

Discuss any insights or benefits the participants had from being able to read someone else's emotions; any benefits they could see happening?

Use the process of the group discussion to help those who may still be having a lot of difficulty understanding the assignment. Throughout sessions, referring back to reading the emotions of others will become part of the natural discussion around situations the participants will discuss.

Some group members are likely to express resistance to the exercises or the concepts in general. Remember, other group members who are becoming successful and seeing the benefits of these exercises are often able to counter group members that are having more difficulty. Questions such as "Do other people feel similarly?" or "Has anyone had a different experience?" help facilitate discussions that can help with all group members' growth.

Keeping an Emotional Response Log

Applying the emotion vocabulary and emotional empathy skills developed in prior sessions to the more difficult task of reading one's own emotions is the summit of the process. At this point, it is vital to acknowledge the progress that the client has made and give full credit for obstacles overcome.

By now, the clients' motivation is apt to be strengthened by a growing sense of mastery and discovery. They have begun to make connections that make life more interesting and rich. A vision of new possibilities may well draw him into the challenge of turning his attention from the feelings of others to his own.

The essential tool for putting the client's own emotions into words is a formal record, the "emotional response log," which he keeps for the duration of the group. Each entry will have three parts:

- The feeling, bodily sensation, or sign of stress that he first becomes aware of. (For many men, this will be the undifferentiated "buzz" of emotional arousal.)

- The context – social situation, conversation, event, or circumstance – in which it occurred. Who is doing what to whom and how does it affect him?
- The identified emotion. Suggest that he go through his vocabulary list to figure out the words that best describe the experience that he is having.

Highlight that there are many good reasons to focus on your emotions, give them a name, and then talk about them. First, naming your feelings affects the part of the brain that controls logic and language, so that when you identify your feelings and put them into words, you get a better sense of control over them. This can help you cope with negative emotions like fear, anger, or sadness. Second, naming your feelings and talking about them is essential for relating well with others; people around you can't always know for certain what you're feeling unless you tell them (Gottman, 2001).

Homework

Clients will spend the next week working on their emotional response log. It is important to have a convenient, easily carried format in which to keep the log. A small notebook, index cards, or a cell phone are possible suggestions. Appendix IV-G presents a possible format for participants to use.

APPENDIX IV-G

Emotional Response Log

Date	Sensation, sign of stress, or feeling	Situation/place/event	Words to describe emotion (Refer to your list)

GROUP: SESSION 5

Review of Homework

Once again, a review of homework begins the session. For those who still are developing the ability to read the emotions of others, some review will still be necessary. Asking other participants to discuss successes they had in reading others emotions, both now and throughout session, is a great way to reinforce this skill in all.

Participants should also return with their emotional response logs for this week. This task typically takes two or more sessions to master, so this week will review and expand on the material presented in the last session.

Have participants discuss experiences from the week and what emotions they were able to pick out from their experiences.

Help them to deepen the experience of their feelings by asking them to identify and label more vulnerable emotions and asking them where in their body they feel that emotion (e.g., stomach, chest, specific musculature). Alternatively, if they are unclear on what emotions they are experiencing or have experienced over the week, start by asking them where in their body they sense the emotion and describe those sensations in as much detail as possible. If a member continues to struggle with labeling a particular emotion, invite other members to reflect on emotions that they may have had associated with the physical sensations being described.

Look for reliance on the old repertoire of emotions, such as anger and "stress" that are typically recorded during first tries at this assignment.

"Don't accept anger at face value" is a useful instruction. If a client can relinquish the empowering experience of anger, he is likely to find vulnerable emotions like fear and hurt underneath.

Men who repeatedly record being "stressed out" should be encouraged to tease apart their unease in search of more specific feelings.

Continue to work with the resistance of group members to the exercises or the concepts in general. Remember, other group members who are becoming successful and seeing the benefits of these exercises are often able to counter group members that are having more difficulty. Questions such as "Do other people feel similarly?" or "Has anyone had a different experience?" help facilitate discussions that can help with all group members' growth.

The Experience of Shame

It is in this stage of therapy that shame is most likely to become an obstacle. The therapist must be particularly supportive, making use of the psychoeducational groundwork already established.

Refer back to the axiom that all emotions are "natural" and "human."

Resistance will be overcome to the extent that the emotional expansion process can be reframed as courageous rather than weak.

Praise participants for being willing to "brave the shame" of violating male socialization taboos.

Discuss the difference between *experiencing* and *expressing* emotions. Being able to experience emotions opens up choices for the client. It does not mean having to show all of his emotions to everyone. In fact, he is now being given back control of his emotional reactions and will be able to choose when and what to express.

Practice

As with any developing skill, practice is the key to making emotional awareness automatic and integrating it into the client's day-to-day life. As sessions continue, feedback from the therapist and other group members can help participants identify the emotions that they have experienced in situations, or even that they are experiencing in the course of the group session. Raising questions of "How did you feel?" and "How do you think she felt?" will continue to reinforce the client's developing skills.

Homework

The same assignment will be repeated for at least the next session, if not the next few sessions. Reminders of working to get underneath the experiences of anger and stress should direct the client in working to uncover their full range of emotions, especially the vulnerable (e.g., fear, sadness) and caring (e.g., tenderness, affection) ones.

GROUP: SESSION 6

Review Homework

As before, check in with participants to review progress in identifying the emotions of others. Spend the appropriate amount of time working to bring the group up to speed on this skill, if needed.

Hopefully the participants' emotional response logs are reflecting a growing awareness of their emotions. Review the logs from the past week.

Ask for instances where participants find that they've uncovered a new emotional experience or were able to keenly identify previously untapped emotions.

Help participants, both those who are and aren't having success, process roadblocks in uncovering emotions.

Discuss benefits or changes that participants are experiencing from being able to identify their emotions.

Continue to work with the resistance of group members to the exercises or the concepts in general. Remember, other group members who are becoming successful and seeing the benefits of these exercises are often able to counter group members that are having more difficulty. Questions such as "Do other people feel similarly?" or "Has anyone had a different experience?" help facilitate discussions that can help with all group members' growth.

Re-administer the NMAS-BF

- See Appendix VI-G.
- With each member of the group, compare the current score to the earlier one and discuss how the score has changed. Look at individual items that were scored differently and discuss.
- Discuss benefits or changes that the client is experiencing from being able to identify their emotions.
- Continue to work with the resistance of the client to the exercises or the concepts in general.

Moving Forward

The client's life itself is likely to provide the most effective feedback. These skills are self-reinforcing for most: men feel empowered and energized as they learn them. Clients become highly motivated when they discover that their emerging empathy, openness, and communication skills reduce conflict and increase harmony in their family lives.

Deeper Issues

As the client becomes more emotionally self-aware, he will start to make connections to other problems, and the relevance of other issues are likely to surface. The conversations of the group will turn from understanding and moving beyond a state of Normative Male Alexithymia to conversations about the difficulties in participants' lives. The therapist simply follows this process as it leads into deeper areas, and directs the clients' application of their emerging emotional skills to work on them.

APPENDIX VI-G

Normative Male Alexithymia Scale-Brief Form

DIRECTIONS: Please use the scale below to indicate the extent to which you personally agree or disagree with each statement. There are no right or wrong responses.

1	2	3	4	5	6	7
Strongly Disagree	Disagree	Slightly Disagree	Neutral or Undecided	Slightly Agree	Agree	Strongly Agree

1. I don't like to talk with others about my feelings.
2. It is difficult for me to reveal my innermost feelings, even to close friends.
3. I feel comfortable expressing my affection to family members and friends.
4. I have difficulty telling others that I care about them.
5. When someone close to me hurts my feelings, I am able to tell them that I am hurt.
6. If someone asks how I am feeling, I typically say what I am not feeling (e.g., "not too bad").

Scoring Instructions: To obtain the total score (mean item score), reverse the scoring of reverse- scored items, and take the mean. Reverse-scored items = 3, 5.

Interpretation of Scores:

Scores can range from low (1) to high (7). The NMAS-BF was not subjected to a clinical assessment to determine cut-off values, as was the TAS-20, so we recommend using the following scheme (using values reported in the validation study) to interpret scores:

Moderately High: Mean plus one standard deviation = 5.36

Very High: Mean plus two standard deviations = 6.68

NOTES

1. For group therapy, the initial intake should be done on an individual basis, which will likely include determining if the client is appropriate for group.
2. It is unusual for a man to come in complaining of difficulty in expressing emotions. Frequently, the visit has been instigated, at least in part, by the client's wife or intimate partner; she typically is the one who has identified his emotional constriction as a problem.
3. Normative Male Alexithymia has been theorized to relate to these clinical syndromes in that they are thought to be the result of maladaptive coping strategies the man has developed in lieu of an ability to verbally process his emotions and seek social support.
4. Include any state statutes regarding the mandatory reporting laws (e.g., child and elder abuse), and limitations of confidentiality based upon the states

statues of duty to protect or duty to warn. Please refer to your state's relevant legal code and all professional ethical guidelines.
5. For group therapy, outline the limitations of confidentiality and the legally non-binding agreement of confidentiality of group participants other than the therapist.
6. Depending on your sense of the group, you may want end at different lengths of time (we suggest between one and five minutes). You want to give enough time for those participants without a fuller lexicon to come up with a few, but not so long as to frustrate those who cannot name more than a few.

CHAPTER NINE

The Efficacy of Alexithymia Reduction Treatment: A Pilot Study[1]

Ronald F. Levant, Margaret J. Halter, Eric W. Hayden, and Christine M. Williams

INTRODUCTION

Levant and colleagues (Levant, 2001; Levant & Kelly, 1989; Levant & Kopecky, 1995) developed a brief psychoeducational intervention designed to remediate Normative Male Alexithymia, which is named Alexithymia Reduction Treatment (ART). Recently, Levant et al. (2008) used this prior work to develop a group treatment manual for ART. ART addresses the role of emotions in behavioral health and the socio-cultural reasons for some individuals having difficulty navigating their emotional experience (particularly traditionally raised men). Participants are guided through exercises in the therapy session and through homework that help them become more aware of their emotional experiences, learn how to interpret, react to, and cope with their emotions, and interact with others on an emotional level. ART consists of six sessions, each of which has homework assignments.

The aim of the present pilot research project was to assess the efficacy of ART in remediating Normative Male Alexithymia and modifying dysfunctional traditional male role attitudes and behaviors, including willingness to seek psychological help. This is the first time that ART has been subjected to such a test. A quasi-experimental design was used.

The investigators hypothesized that after receiving ART, the participants in the Treatment Group would report lower scores on a measure of normative male alexithymia, less endorsement of traditional masculinity ideology, and greater self-reported willingness to seek psychological help. The investigators further hypothesized that the Treatment as Usual (TAU) group would show none of these changes.

DOI: 10.4324/9781003378518-13

METHOD

Participants

Inclusion criteria for this pilot study included the ability to give informed consent, read and write English, and be enrolled as a patient at one of the two sites used for the study. The Treatment Group was drawn from the University of Akron Counseling, Testing and Career Center (CTCC). The CTCC offers free, comprehensive psychological services to currently enrolled students at the University of Akron. Study participants were enrolled in a ten-session group aimed at understanding self and others in order to learn how to manage relationships more effectively, in which ART was the treatment for the first six sessions of the group. Of the six participants, five identified themselves as European American and one identified himself as Latino. Their ages ranged from 18 to 33, with an average age of 24. One participant reported having a gay sexual orientation, the others reported their orientation as heterosexual; three reported being single, one was divorced, and two reported being involved in serious dating relationships. Five reported having a high school diploma or GED, and one reported having a bachelor's degree. Their modal income was between $20,000 and $40,000 a year. In terms of religion, one identified himself as Jewish, one as Christian, one as Pagan, one as agnostic, and two as atheist.

The Treatment as Usual (TAU) group was drawn from the Partial Hospitalization Program (PHP) at Akron General Medical Center (AGMC). The PHP provides a day treatment format primarily for patients who have severe depression and are capable of participating in a group setting. During the course of a six-hour day, patients attend groups focused on goal setting, psychotherapy, recreational therapy, psychoeducational therapy (e.g., psychopharmacology and diagnosis understanding), and art therapy. The length of stay varies from approximately five to ten days. This group was chosen based on the fact that these individuals were also in regular group therapy and would approximate qualities of those participating in group therapy at the University of Akron. All seven participants identified themselves as European American. Their ages ranged from 21 to 54, with an average age of 39. All reported their sexual orientation as heterosexual; four reported being married or partnered, one reported being single, one was divorced, and one reported being involved in a serious dating relationship. Four reported having a high school diploma or GED, two reported having a bachelor's degree, and one reported having a master's degree. The modal income was between $80,000 and $100,000 a year. In terms of religion, six identified themselves as Christian, and one identified himself as agnostic.

Procedure

The participants were given an oral and written explanation of the study and asked if they would like to be included. If receptive, informed consent was obtained, and the participant was made aware that his participation was completely voluntary and that he could withdraw from the study at any time. The participants completed the instruments described below immediately prior to beginning treatment and upon completion of the course of the six-session ART intervention (for the Treatment Group) and at discharge (for the Treatment as Usual group). The usual time necessary to complete the questionnaires was about 30 minutes.

Participants in the Treatment Group at the University of Akron Counseling, Testing, and Career Center received a manualized psychoeducational group treatment, which was administered in the first six sessions of their therapy group (Levant et al., 2008). ART consists of six sessions, each of which has homework assignments: (1) Male Emotion Socialization; (2) Developing a Vocabulary for Emotions; (3) Learning to Read the Emotions of Others; (4) Keeping an Emotional Response Log; (5) Practice; and (6) Moving to Deeper Issues. Participants completed a short series of self-report instruments at the beginning of therapy and again after the sixth and final session of ART. ART was provided by a licensed psychologist and a pre-doctoral psychology intern. The group leaders who provided the intervention participated in a training program conducted by Levant, which included several readings, a lecture, watching a videotape, discussion of the forgoing, and study of the treatment manual.

The Treatment as Usua group at AGMC received the program's usual group therapy treatments without the manualized psychoeducational interventions. Participants in this group were also asked to complete a short series of self-report instruments when they were admitted and again at the time of discharge.

Measures

Demographic Questionnaire

A brief demographic questionnaire was used to gather data on race/ethnicity, age, sexual orientation, relationship status, highest degree completed, family/household income, self-rated socioeconomic status, and religion.

Normative Male Alexithymia Scale

To measure Normative Male Alexithymia the investigators used the Normative Male Alexithymia Scale (NMAS) (Levant et al., 2006). The NMAS is a 20-item inventory designed to assess normative male alexithymia (e.g., "I am often confused about what emotion I am feeling.") Participants answer questions about their own experience of emotions using a Likert-type format (1 = *strongly disagree*, 7 = *strongly agree*), with higher scores indicating higher levels of alexithymia. Exploratory and confirmatory factor analysis indicated that the NMAS consisted of a single 20-item factor. Scores on the NMAS displayed very good internal consistency ($\alpha = .92$ for men and $\alpha = .93$ for women) and test–retest reliability ($r = .91$ for men and $r = .82$ for women) over a one to two month period. Results of analyses of sex differences, relations of the NMAS with other instruments, and its incremental validity in predicting scores on a measure of masculinity ideology provided evidence supporting the validity of the scale.

Male Role Norms Inventory-Revised

To assess participants' endorsement of traditional masculinity ideology, the investigators used the Male Role Norms Inventory-Revised (MRNI-R) (Levant et al., 2007). This measure assesses traditional masculinity ideology and beliefs about the importance of adhering to culturally defined standards for masculine behavior. The revised version of the MRNI-R is a 53-item measure with items rated on a seven-point Likert-type scale (1 = *strongly disagree*; 7 = *strongly agree*), with higher scores indicating higher levels of endorsement of traditional masculinity ideology. Seven subscales assess individuals' endorsement of different facets of traditional masculinity ideology, including: Avoidance of Femininity (eight items, e.g., "A man should prefer watching action movies to reading romantic novels."); Fear and Hatred of Homosexuals (ten items, e.g., "Homosexuals should never marry."); Extreme Self-Reliance (seven items, e.g., "Men should not borrow money from friends or family members."); Dominance (seven items, e.g., "A man should always be the boss."); Non-Relational Sexuality (six items, e.g., "A man should always be ready for sex."); and Restrictive Emotionality (eight items, e.g., "Men should not be too quick to tell others that they care about them."). A total scale score may also be obtained through the averaging of scores on all 53 items. Adequate coefficient alpha reliabilities were found for the MRNI-R total and its subscales, ranging from .73 to .96 (Levant et al., 2007). Results indicate good convergent validity through the significant inter-correlations of the MRNI-R with the Male Role Attitudes Scale, Conformity to Masculine Norms Inventory, the Gender Role Conflict Scale, and the Normative Male Alexithymia Scale. It also showed good discriminant validity in that strong positive correlations with the Personal Attributes Questionnaire were not found (Levant et al., 2010).

Attitudes toward Seeking Professional Psychological Help Scale (ATSPPH-Short Form)

The ATSPPH-Short Form (Fischer & Farina, 1995) is comprised of ten items asking about the respondent's attitudes toward psychological services (e.g.,

"A person with an emotional problem is not likely to solve it alone; he or she is likely to solve it with professional help."). Answers are recorded in a Likert-type format consisting of four alternatives: *agree*, *partly agree*, *partly disagree*, and *disagree*. "Straight" items, expressing positive help-seeking attitudes, are coded 4, 3, 2, 1; reverse-scored items, expressing negative help-seeking attitudes, are coded 1, 2, 3, 4. Scores range from 10 to 40, with higher scores representing more positive attitudes toward professional psychological help-seeking. Fischer and Farina found support for the reliability and validity of this version of the ATSPPH. The correlation between the long and short versions of the scale was .87. The internal consistency reliability was sufficient in the shortened measure (Cronbach's alpha = .84), and test–retest reliability was .80 after a one-month interval. Factor analysis indicated that the measure consisted of one general factor. Women reported significantly more favorable attitudes than men (Fischer & Farina).

RESULTS

As can be seen from Table 9.1, participants in the ART group demonstrated significant reductions in Normative Male Alexithymia on the NMAS and the endorsement of traditional masculinity ideology on the MRNI-R (Dominance, Restrictive Emotionality, and Total). In contrast the Treatment as Usual group did not demonstrate significant reductions in any of these variables from pre-test to post-test. Neither group showed significant change in attitudes toward seeking professional psychological help on the ATSPPH.

DISCUSSION

The limitations of the pilot study include the fact that the sample size was small, that the treatment and comparison groups were drawn from two very different clinical settings, that the length and intensity of the interventions provided to the two groups differed, and that there were demographic differences between the two groups; hence the results need to be viewed with great caution. The significant findings could just as likely be due to the differences in the settings and participants as to the differences between ART and TAU.

Even with these limitations, ART demonstrated changes in two of the three target areas: Reducing Normative Male Alexithymia and reducing the endorsement of traditional male role norms. Hence, there is an indication that ART may have efficacy.

TABLE 9.1 Means, Standard Deviations, and T-Tests Comparing Pre- and Post-Test Means for the Treatment and Treatment as Usual Comparison Groups

Measure	ART (N = 6)				Treatment as Usual (N = 7)			
	Mean	SD	t^a	p	Mean	SD	T^b	p
NMAS-T1	4.26	1.45			4.17	1.50		
NMAS-T2	3.35	.89	2.54	.05	3.43	1.14	1.93	.10
MRNI-R-Subscales								
AVF-T1	3.12	1.77			3.25	1.05		
AVF-T2	2.94	1.65	1.63	.17	3.00	1.42	1.10	.32
FHH-T1	2.28	1.46			3.20	1.02		
FHH-T2	2.17	1.38	1.47	.20	3.27	1.01	-.36	.73
SR-T1	3.36	1.34			3.53	1.07		
SR-T2	3.26	1.31	.93	.39	3.16	1.12	.85	.43
AGG-T1	4.02	1.33			3.65	1.33		
AGG-T2	3.81	1.12	1.70	.15	3.90	.96	-1.28	.25
DOM-T1	2.38	1.29			2.53	1.47		
DOM-T2	2.19	1.21	3.16	.03	2.45	.89	.20	.85
NRS-T1	2.28	.99			2.76	1.47		
NRS-T2	2.11	.87	1.94	.11	2.71	1.39	.23	.83
REMO-T1	2.17	1.08			2.48	.77		
REMO-T2	1.98	.95	3.00	.03	2.30	.87	.60	.57
MRNI-R Total-T1	2.78	1.15			3.07	.96		
MRNI-R Total-T2	2.61	1.06	2.85	.04	2.98	.85	.36	.73
ATSPPH-T1	23.17	4.71			26.14	2.28		
ATSPPH-T2	21.83	4.58	1.66	.16	27.25	2.07	-1.54	.18

Legend: T1 = pre-test; T2 = post-test; NMAS = Normative Male Alexithymia Scale; MRNI-R = Male Role Norms Inventory-Revised; AVF = Avoidance of Femininity MRNI-R subscale; FHH = Fear and Hatred of Homosexuals MRNI-R subscale; SR = Extreme Self-Reliance MRNI-R subscale; AGG = Aggression MRNI-R subscale; Dom = Dominance MRNI-R subscale; NRS = Non-Relational Attitudes toward Sex MRNI-R subscale; REMO = Restrictive Emotionality MRNI-R subscale; MRNI-R Total = Male Role Norms Inventory-Revised Total Score; ATSPPH = Attitudes toward Seeking Professional Psychological Help Scale.
a Comparing Pre- and Post-Test Means for the Treatment Group.
b Comparing Pre- and Post-Test Means for the Treatment As Usual Comparison Group.

Another study, conducted in Pakistan, bolsters this conclusion. Akram and Arshad (2022) tested the efficacy of ART as an online group intervention with male university students ($n = 20$). The participants were assigned to a treatment group ($n = 10$) or wait-list control group ($n = 10$). The participants were assigned to the treatment and wait-list control group based on their availability to attend the therapeutic sessions; thus, this was another quasi-experimental clinical trial. The treatment group then received ART while the wait-list control received no treatment at that time. The results showed a significant reduction in the treatment group participants' alexithymia, as well as their depression and anxiety. These changes were not found in the wait-list control group.

Levant and Dr. Mike Parent are planning a randomized controlled study of the efficacy of ART, using the online asynchronous intervention system TinCat, developed by Dr. Parent. Traditional counseling services require that clients and therapists have matching available times for mental health services. Because mental health services constitute jobs for those providing the services, most of the available therapist times are during the normal working day. Most clients have normal work and/or school schedules, which overlap completely with the working schedules of therapists. Thus, the need to temporally couple therapist and client available times represents a major barrier to accessing traditional mental health services. This barrier is further exacerbated by challenges in going to sessions in person (e.g., a one-hour therapy session in the middle of the day may require a half hour drive each way, necessitating taking multiple hours off of school or work) and by challenges in technology for synchronous telehealth services (e.g., net connectivity issues, telehealth platform outages, audio/video issues). TinCat provides accessible mental health intervention by enabling interventions to de-couple from temporal synchronization.

In TinCat intervention, therapy sessions are recorded by a therapist and sent to the client online, to be viewed (and re-viewed) at any time. Sessions are limited to seven to ten minutes (consistent with research on time limits for information intake). Specific strategies are used to ensure that clients know that TinCat intervention videos are made specially for them. For example, TinCat procedures require the name of the client to be used at least four times in a video and require at least one specific reference to material covered in a prior session that is unique to that client. These steps ensure that individuals enrolled in TinCat are aware that their therapist is working directly with them, and the sessions are not pre-recorded. These steps facilitate the development of a parasocial relationship (i.e., a unidirectional relationship in which the client feels seen and valued by the therapist). Research has demonstrated that parasocial relationships are powerful influences on health behaviors. The demonstrated efficacy of the TinCat model disrupts the traditional notion of the therapy relationship in that it replicates the importance of feeling seen and understood on the part of the client, without the need for that relationship to exist only during inefficient temporal coupling of sessions.

Prior research demonstrated the efficacy of the TinCat model in providing manualized CBT for depression to sexual and gender minority adults enrolled in the pilot study. Individuals enrolled in both the intervention (TinCat personalized treatment) and the control group (non-personalized videos that went through the manualized CBT treatment) improved during the course of treatment, but TinCat intervention group participants retained all gains at the four-week follow up whereas the control group regressed to baseline levels.

The planned study will use the TinCat method to apply ART to college men. College men are reluctant to engage in help-seeking, and men who experience alexithymia are particularly reluctant to engage in mental health services.

Finding ART efficacious could improve the process and outcome of psychotherapy for men who are alexithymic, as well as alexithymic patients struggling with medical illnesses (Beresnevaite, 2000; Courtenay, 2000). Thus, this would open up an area for future research that investigates the effects of this brief psychoeducational intervention on the process and outcome of psychotherapy for alexithymic men who are being treated for both mental and physical conditions. Finding the program efficacious could encourage the development of treatments and preventive interventions tailored to the gender-specific needs of boys and men.

NOTE

1. Chapter 9, entire chapter. Adapted with permission from Levant, R. F., Halter, M. J., Hayden, E., & Williams, C. (2009). The efficacy of alexithymia reduction treatment: A pilot study, *Journal of Men's Studies, 17*(1) 75–84. doi:10.3149/jms.1701.x Reprinted by permission from Sage Publications.

REFERENCES

Addis, M. E., & Mahalik, J. R. (2003). Men, masculinity, and the contexts of help-seeking. *American Psychologist, 58*, 5–14. https://doi.org/10.1037/0003-066X.58.1.5

Akram, A., & Arshad, T. (2022) Alexithymia reduction treatment: A pilot quasi-experimental study for remediation of alexithymia and its consequent effects on the general mental health of university students. *Counselling and Psychotherapy Research, 22*(4), 902–912. https://doi.org/10.1002/capr.12571

Berger, J. M., Levant, R. F., McMillan, K. K., Kelleher, W., & Sellers, A. (2005). Impact of gender role conflict, traditional masculinity ideology, alexithymia, and age on men's attitudes toward psychological help seeking. *Psychology of Men and Masculinity, 6,* 73–78. https://doi.org/10.1037/1524-9220.6.1.73

Beresnevaite, M. (2000). Exploring the benefits of group psychotherapy in reducing alexithymia in coronary heart disease patients: An exploratory study. *Psychotherapy and Psychosomatics, 69,* 117–122. https://doi.org/10.1159/000012378

Brody, L. R., & Hall, J. A. (1993). Gender and emotion. In M. Lewis & J. M. Haviland (Eds.), *Handbook of emotions* (pp. 447–460). New York: Guilford Press.

Brown, L. (2005). The neglect of lesbian, gay, bisexual, and transgendered clients. In J. C. Norcross, L. E. Beutler, & R. F. Levant (Eds.), *Evidence-based practices in mental health: Debate and dialogue on the fundamental questions* (pp. 346–352). Washington, DC: APA.

Buck, R. (1977). Nonverbal communication of affect in preschool children: Relationships with personality and skin conductance. *Journal of Personality and Social Psychology, 35,* 225–236. https://doi.org/10.1037/0022-3514.35.4.225

Courtenay, W. H. (2000). Behavioral factors associated with disease, injury, and death among men: Evidence and implications for prevention. *The Journal of Men's Studies, 9,* 81–142. https://doi.org/10.3149/jms.0901.81

Dunn, J., Bretherton, I., & Munn, P. (1987). Conversations about feeling states between mothers and their young children. *Developmental Psychology, 23,* 132–139. https://doi.org/10.1037/0012-1649.23.1.132

Fischer, E. H., & Farina, A. (1995). Attitudes toward seeking professional psychological help: A shortened form and considerations for research. *Journal of College Student Development, 36,* 368–373. https://doi.org/10.1037/t05375-000

Fivush, R. (1989). Exploring sex differences in the emotional content of mother-child conversations about the past. *Sex Roles, 20,* 11–12. https://doi.org/10.1007/BF00288079

Haviland, J. J., & Malatesta, C. Z. (1981). The development of sex differences in nonverbal signals: Fallacies, facts, and fantasies. In C. Mayo & N. M. Henly (Eds.), *Gender and non-verbal behavior* (pp. 183–208). New York: Springer-Verlag.

Lamb, M. E. (1977). The development of mother-infant and father-infant attachments in the second year of life. *Developmental Psychology, 13,* 637–648. https://doi.org/10.1037/0012-1649.13.6.637

Lamb, M. E., Owen, M. J., & Chase-Lansdale, L. (1979). The father daughter relationship: Past, present, and future. In C. B. Knopp & M. Kirkpatrick (Eds.), *Becoming female.* New York: Plenum.

Langlois, J. H., & Downs, A. C. (1980). Mothers, fathers, and peers as socialization agents of sex-type play behaviors in young children. *Child Development, 51,* 1237–1247. https://doi.org/10.2307/1129566

Levant, R. F. (1992). Toward the reconstruction of masculinity. *Journal of Family Psychology, 5,* 379–402. https://doi.org/10.1037/0893-3200.5.3-4.379

Levant, R. F. (1995). Toward the reconstruction of masculinity. In R. F. Levant & W. S. Pollack (Eds.), *A new psychology of men* (pp. 229–251). New York: Basic Books.

Levant, R. F. (1998). Desperately seeking language: Understanding, assessing, and treating normative male alexithymia. In W. Pollack & R. F. Levant (Eds.), *New psychotherapy for men* (pp. 35–56). New York: John Wiley.

Levant, R. F. (2001). Desperately seeking language: Understanding, assessing, and treating normative male alexithymia. In W. Pollack & R. F. Levant (Eds.), *The new handbook of psychotherapy and counseling with men: A comprehensive guide to settings, problems, and treatment approaches* (Vol. 1 & 2, pp. 424–443). San Francisco: Jossey-Bass.

Levant, R. F., Good, G. E., Cook, S., O'Neil, J., Smalley, K. B., Owen, K. A., et al. (2006). Validation of the normative male alexithymia scale: Measurement of a gender-linked syndrome. *Psychology of Men & Masculinity, 7*, 212–224. https://doi.org/10.1037/1524-9220.7.4.212

Levant, R. F., Halter, M. J., Hayden, E. W., & Williams, C. M. (2009). The efficacy of alexithymia reduction treatment: A pilot study. *The Journal of Men's Studies, 17*(1), 75–84. https://doi-org.ezproxy.uakron.edu:2443/10.3149/jms.1701.75

Levant, R. F., & Kelly, J. (1989). *Between father and child: How to become the kind of father you want to be.* New York: Viking.

Levant, R. F., & Kopecky, G. (1995). *Masculinity reconstructed.* New York: Plume.

Levant, R. F., Rankin, T. J., Williams, C. M., Hasan, N. T., & Smalley, K. B. (2010). Evaluation of the factor structure and construct validity of scores on the Male Role Norms Inventory—Revised (MRNI-R). *Psychology of Men & Masculinity, 11*(1), 25. https://doi.org/10.1037/a0017637

Levant, R. F., & Richmond, K. (2007). A review of research on masculinity ideologies using the male role norms inventory. *Journal of Men's Studies, 15*, 130–146. *https://doi.org/10.3149/jms.1502.130*

Levant, R. F., & Silverstein, L. B. (2005). Gender is neglected in both evidence based practices and treatment as usual. In J. C. Norcross, L. E. Beutler, & R. F. Levant (Eds.), *Evidence-based practices in mental health: Debate and dialogue on the fundamental questions* (pp. 338–345). Washington, DC: APA.

Levant, R. F., Smalley, K. B., Aupont, M., House, A., Richmond, K., & Noronha, D. (2007). Validation of the male role norms inventory- revised. *Journal of Men's Studies, 15,* 85–100.

Levant, R. F., & Williams, C. (2007). Sex differences in alexithymia: A Meta-Analysis. (submitted to refereed journal).

Levant, R. F., Williams, C., & Hayden, E. (2008). Alexithymia Reduction Treatment (ART): A manual for a brief psycho-educational intervention for treating normative male alexithymia, group therapy format. Unpublished Manual: University of Akron Lever, J. R. (1976). Sex differences in the games children play. *Social Problems, 23,* 478–487. https://doi.org/10.2307/799857

Levant, R. F., Williams, C., Smalley, K. B., & Richmond, K. (2007). Reliability and discriminant and convergent construct validity for the MRNI-R. (under review at referred journal).

Maccoby, E. E. (1994). The role of gender identity and gender constancy in sex-differentiated development. In B. Puka (Ed.), *Caring voices and women's moral frames: Gilligan's view* (pp. 295–310). New York & London: Garland Publishing.

Mahalik, J. R., Lagan, H. D., & Morrison, J. A. (2006). Health behaviors and masculinity in Kenyan and U.S. male college students. *Psychology of Men & Masculinity, 7,* 191–202. https://doi.org/10.1037/1524-9220.7.4.191

McCallum, M. Piper, W. E., Ogrodniczuk, J. S., & Joyce, A, S. (2003). Relationships among psychological mindedness, alexithymia, and outcome in four forms of short-term psychotherapy. *Psychology and Psychotherapy: Theory, Research and Practice, 76,* 133–144. https://doi.org/10.1348/147608303765951177

Norcross, J. C., Beutler, L. E., & Levant, R. F. (2005). *Evidence-based practices in mental health: Debate and dialogue on the fundamental questions.* Washington, DC: APA.

Ogrodniczuk, J. S., Piper, W. E., & Joyce, A. S. (2004). Alexithymia as a predictor of residual symptoms in depressed patients who respond to short-term psychotherapy. *American Journal of Psychotherapy, 82,* 469–473.

O'Neil, J. M., Good G. E., & Holmes, S. (1995). Fifteen years of theory and research on men's gender role conflict: New paradigms for empirical research. In W. Pollack & R. F. Levant (Eds.), *New psychotherapy for men* (pp. 164–206). New York: John Wiley.

Paley, V. G. (1984). *Boys and girls: Superheroes in the doll corner.* Chicago: University of Chicago Press.

Pleck, J. H. (1981). *The myth of masculinity.* Cambridge, MA: MIT Press.

Pleck, J. H. (1995). The gender role strain paradigm: An update. In R. F. Levant & W. S. Pollack (Eds.), *A new psychology of men* (pp. 11–32). New York: Basic Books.

Pollack, W. S. (1998). The trauma of Oedipus: Toward a new psychoanalytic psychotherapy for men. In W. S. Pollack & R. F. Levant (Eds.), *New psychotherapy for men* (pp. 13–34). Hoboken, NJ: John Wiley & Sons.

Siegal, M. (1987). Are sons and daughters treated more differently by fathers than by mothers? *Developmental Review, 7,* 183–209. https://doi.org/10.1016/0273-2297(87)90012-8

Sue, S., & Zane, N. (2005). How well do both evidence-based practices and treatment as usual satisfactorily address the various dimensions of diversity. In J. C. Norcross, L. E. Beutler, & R. F. Levant (Eds.), *Evidence-based practices in mental health: Debate and dialogue on the fundamental questions* (pp. 329–374). Washington, DC: APA.

PART IV
Case Studies

Finally, we present two case studies that illustrate the use of ART, first in individual therapy, and the second in couple therapy. Both cases were treated by Levant, who in general worked from a Bowen family systems model.

CHAPTER TEN

The Man Who Felt Nothing about His Impending Fatherhood

Ronald F. Levant

To give the reader an idea of how this approach works for men, we present a case study of a man with alexithymia treated using Alexithymia Reduction Treatment.[1] This case study has been made into a teaching videotape in which an actor plays the role of the client and is available from: www.psychotherapy .net/video/psychotherapy-men-ron-levant

REASON FOR REFERRAL

Raymond called for an appointment because he "felt nothing" about the fact that he and his wife were expecting their first child. His wife's distress over his lack of feelings, and his concern about her feelings, were the two primary motivators in his decision to seek therapy. Apart from the fact that his wife was pregnant and he thought he "should" feel something about that, Raymond did not find it particularly odd that he "felt nothing." He usually felt nothing. The last time he cried was when his dog was killed by a car. That was ten years ago.

PERSONAL DATA

Raymond and his wife, Caroline, are both college-educated. He works as a financial consultant and has had a satisfactory, unexceptional work history, with no problems in his profession. His wife works also, but her career has always taken second place to his, in part because his work is largely responsible for the family income. Theirs is essentially a traditional marriage in which he is the main

DOI: 10.4324/9781003378518-15

"breadwinner." They met several years after college, are both 40 years old, and have been married for 15 years. They postponed starting a family because job moves earlier in Raymond's career made them feel too "unsettled." Raymond seems neat, well-groomed, and well-spoken. He has an all-business manner – competent, unemotional, and not playful; he is not one to "schmooz" or treat things lightly. Although he does not seem clinically depressed, he comes across with a somewhat dejected air.

FAMILY HISTORY

Raymond is the oldest child and only son of a newspaper publisher in a small Midwestern town, and his wife, a full-time homemaker. He has twin sisters. His mother is widowed. His father, who was substantially older than his mother, died of heart disease in his late 60s. Throughout Raymond's childhood, his father seemed emotionally disengaged from the family, but was very involved with his newspaper and with community affairs. His home was open to community leaders until late in the evening, leaving little time for his family.

Raymond remains involved, in a highly responsible way, with his family of origin; his mother lives nearby and one of his sisters is divorced and has a disabled child, and he contributes substantially to their support.

DIAGNOSIS

Normative Male Alexithymia as a diagnosis will not be found in the *Diagnostic and Statistical Manual of Mental Disorders* (DSM). Since therapy is most often paid for by some form of health insurance, a DSM diagnosis is necessary to communicate with the third-party payor. In my clinical experience, DSM diagnoses may or may not have much to do with the therapy; sometimes they are very relevant, and other times they are not so relevant.

In this case, I considered somatization disorder, which I ruled out because even though the patient tended to somaticize his vulnerable emotions, he did not meet the specific criteria for that diagnosis. On balance, I felt that the multiaxial diagnosis summarized below fit the patient reasonably well, though it did not have as much bearing on therapy as the non-DSM diagnosis of Normative Male Alexithymia.

- Axis I: Adjustment disorder, with mixed emotional features, anxiety, and depressed mood.
- Axis II: Patient has no Axis II diagnoses.

- Axis III: Apart from the tendency to somaticize his vulnerable emotions, the patient has no medical illnesses.
- Axis IV: Patient's problems are with his "primary support group" (i.e., his wife).
- Axis V: I gave the patient a global assessment of function score (GAF) of 65, which indicates mild symptomatology.

THE COURSE OF THERAPY

This case was somewhat unusual in that Raymond came specifically for treatment of emotional numbness and did not have to be "sold" on the need for psychoeducational therapy to address his alexithymia.

The treatment involved 15 sessions over the course of five months. We met weekly as we did the work of Sessions 1 through 4. Raymond worked hard during this period and became more able to identify his emotions and put them into words. But after that, events (business trips, holidays) intervened, and sessions tended to be several weeks apart. This is not unusual; in fact, it is often useful to space sessions out in the middle stages of therapy in order to put more emphasis on the client's own work on issues outside therapy, and to meet less frequently as therapy tapers off.

Raymond said at the outset that he thought that a lot of his problems had to do with his father. His father was 11 years older than his mother, was 38 when Raymond was born, and had died of a heart attack 13 years prior to the onset of therapy. Raymond believed that his father had a great life as an Air Force officer during World War II – a life that he had to leave behind when he married and started a family, and one that he seemed to miss greatly. His father was a tail gunner, and said he never felt more alive than when he was on a mission, "sitting in the butt end of a bomber, two seconds from death," as he often put it. Because of his father's self-absorption and detachment, Raymond was always unsure of his father's feelings about him. And yet he yearned to get closer. For example, Raymond's lifelong hobby was participating in Scottish rites and learning about his Scottish ancestry, an activity in which he had earlier hoped he could involve his father. The first time I saw Raymond display emotions openly was when he spoke of how he had always wanted to see his dad in a kilt, carrying a set of bagpipes.

As therapy progressed, Raymond's initial detachment about his father turned to curiosity. Raymond discovered he had many questions he wanted to ask his father, so we constructed a therapeutic ritual in which he would write down the questions that he had for his father on 3" x 5" cards. I also suggested digging out old family photos to stimulate his memories. His initial response to these tasks was to get very angry that his father "just wasn't there." He later talked of how, when his father needed him after his first heart attack, he decided he was too busy to visit. In describing this event, he said "It's a family curse. I come from a long line of uncaring fathers."

The therapy deepened on a trip to visit his father's grave. He described the experience as "raw emotion." His sadness poured out of him, as he stood alone at his father's headstone, reading through his cards filled with unanswered questions.

He was later able to locate an old friend of his father, Henry, who remembered the day Raymond was born. Henry said that that was the only time he saw Raymond's father cry. We can never know how accurate Henry's recollection is, but that is not the point. Raymond was able to use this information to be able to feel for the first time in his life that maybe his father really did care about him after all. With this shift Raymond then was able to begin to address a lifelong sense of shame, which stemmed in no small measure from his relationship with his father.

Having made progress in addressing his sense of shame and recapturing his ability to tune into and verbalize his emotional life, Raymond began to experience some strong feelings about his expectant fatherhood – fear, worry, and anxiety. He began to worry about whether the baby was going to be all right, given his wife's age. He also investigated some obscure genetic diseases that ran in families of Scottish descent. I encouraged him to address his worries directly, by attending one of his wife's visits to the obstetrician. He did so, and was reassured about the baby's health, and also heard the baby's heartbeat. His fear then turned to joy and excitement. We terminated one month before the baby was due. I got a postcard from him two months later.

Ron, the baby was 2 weeks late. But he's a big guy, 8 lbs 13 oz And he definitely looks Scottish.

NOTE

1. Chapter 10, adapted with permission from Levant, R. F. (2000). A quarter century of psychotherapy. In J. Shay & J. Wheelis (Eds.), *Odysseys in psychotherapy* (pp. 187–208). New York: Irvington Press.

CHAPTER ELEVEN

The "Both/And" Approach to Treating a Postmodern Couple[1]

Ronald F. Levant and Louise B. Silverstein

This chapter arises out of an ongoing collaboration in which we are working to combine family systems theory and gender theory into an integrated approach to couples and family therapy. Family systems theory (Bowen, 1978; Kerr & Bowen, 1988) has emphasized the reciprocal nature of relationship processes, minimizing gender differences in communication styles and expectations about power and privilege. Feminist theory, in contrast, has made gender politics the focus of treatment and has minimized the systemic nature of relationships. Our efforts carry forward the pioneering "both/and" approach of Goldner (1988), who integrated feminist and family systems theory in her work with intimate partner violence. However, we prefer to refer to *gender theory* rather than feminist theory because our thinking also integrates the perspective of the new psychology of men (Levant & Pollack, 1995). Thus, we integrate what is known about gender differences (including masculine gender socialization and role strain) with a grasp of relationships as "emotional systems." Integrating these two theoretical paradigms provides couples with the tools for getting "unstuck" from even the most intractable relationship crises. To date, we have used this approach only with White, heterosexual, middle-class couples. In order for it to be useful for a wide range of couples, issues of immigration, ethnicity, racism, class bias, and homophobia would need to be incorporated in the same way that gender ideology has been addressed in the current model.

DOI: 10.4324/9781003378518-16

THE BUILDING BLOCKS OF OUR INTEGRATED APPROACH

This is a multiphasic approach, and we outline it briefly below. Although we describe three phases of treatment, it is not a sequential or linear process. These phases can occur simultaneously and interact with each other in complex ways.

Phase 1: Learning To "Think Gender": Educate the Couple to Not Take Things Personally

When the person we love most in the world does not respond in the way that we hoped he or she would, we might feel rejected, neglected, and even unloved. However, when we begin to see this person's behavior as the result of the past 3,000 years of gender socialization, it is sometimes easier to feel less personally betrayed. Our approach teaches couples to view their partner's upsetting behaviors as "gender-based disappointments" that are the result of a historical and cultural framework. This reframing allows the injured partner to begin to feel less personally betrayed and can defuse relationship conflict.

Treat the Man's Normative Alexithymia

Levant and Kopecky (1995/1996) described how traditional masculine gender role socialization leads to the development of Normative Male Alexithymia, that is, the inability to discern one's own emotions and put them into words. We use a psychoeducational approach, called Alexithymia Reduction Treatment, to help men overcome alexithymia and to develop emotional self-awareness.

Help the Woman Let Go of the Responsibility for the Couple's Emotional Life

Traditional feminine gender role socialization trains women to feel that they are responsible for managing the emotions of the couple. Again, we use a psychoeducational approach to help women relinquish sole responsibility for the emotional life of the couple. Explaining the dynamics of pursuing and distancing in marital interaction can also be very helpful here.

Phase 2: Learning to "Think Systems"

Many people believe that if only they could find the "right man" or the "right woman," their marriage would work. People enter most relationships with an unrealistic expectation of how well a spouse should fit their ideal. As real life begins to interfere with one's fantasy of "the perfect marriage," a person tends to blame his or her spouse. The person assumes that he or she has simply married the "wrong" man or woman. Unless this misconception (which is based on what Bowen, 1978, described as "emotional fusion") is corrected, couples tend either to divorce or continue to live together in an atmosphere of blame and dissatisfaction.

Although it is easy to be clear about all the things one's partner does wrong, it is infinitely more difficult to focus on the part that one plays in beginning or maintaining negative relationship patterns. It is very easy to get caught in the "blame game." However, if a person does succeed in acknowledging what he or she contributes to the problem, he or she can then become empowered to change many of the unsatisfying aspects of the relationship.

A central construct in family systems theory is "differentiation of self," which is roughly equivalent to emotional maturity (Bowen, 1978). Individuals with emotional problems have lower degrees of differentiation of Self, which is reflected in their tendency to borrow or lend the Self to others. As a result, behavior for such individuals is *reciprocal – that* is, the behavior of each person in a relationship is dependent on and reinforced by the behavior of the Other(s). Therefore, if one person in a relationship changes, those changes will be felt by the other person, and he or she also will change, automatically. Hence, if even one person in a relationship can increase the ability to focus on the Self, the total amount of conflict decreases. Our approach challenges each member of the couple to stop trying to change the Other and begin to take responsibility for changing the Self. This shift in gaze from Other to Self is a major component of our work.

Phase 3: Family-of-Origin Work

Most people can incorporate some of the principles of Phases 1 and 2 into their relationships. They then may experience a dramatic decrease in conflict and a dramatic increase in the pleasure of their intimate relationships. However, some patterns of relating have developed over many generations and so are extremely difficult to change. For many people, understanding gender issues and the reciprocal nature of patterns of relating is not enough to achieve the kind of self-focus that is necessary for enduring behavior change.

The ways in which people respond to their intimate partners have been established in their families during the very early years of life. Thus, the most effective way of changing those patterns is to return to one's early attachment figures and change the way in which one responds to family members. In Bowen family systems theory it is necessary to rework the original relationships, that is, to practice being a Self in the presence of one's family. Work in the context of the therapeutic relationship is not sufficient.

We suggest that our clients undertake efforts to uncover the patterns of relating that have developed in their families of origin, including those based on gender role socialization. Most systems of therapy teach people to look back into their families to understand what happened to them as children. However, in some approaches one's understanding does not get beyond what one's parents did wrong. This way of thinking about families is not helpful because it institutionalizes our tendency to blame our parents rather than helping one take responsibility for oneself. Unless one can achieve an empathic understanding of one's parents as children in their own families, one usually remains stuck in a pattern of blaming one's spouse. Maintaining a sense of one's self as an innocent victim of evil parents perpetuates a focus on the "sins" of one's partner.

I (RL) will provide an example of family-of-origin work from my own life, showing how I was able to be my Self in my family of origin. I lived in the Boston area as a graduate student and young psychologist, and periodically visited my parents in Oxnard, California. These visits usually devolved very quickly into an angry outburst from my father, which put a severe damper on the visit. Applying Bowen's theory to my own life, I realized I was caught up in a triangle, in which my mother would dote on me, my father would become jealous and lash out at me, and I would react by reverting to the surly adolescent I once was. To detriangle, I deflected my mother's efforts to nurture me, and rerouted them to my dad. So, for example she might ask if I was hungry, and would I like her to make something for me to eat? I would respond: "I am fine, mom, but dad might be hungry. Why don't you see if he would like for you to make something for him to eat." This worked like magic.

A POSTMODERN COUPLE AT AN IMPASSE

The case described in this chapter was treated by RL and is written from his point of view. Barbara, age 38, is a highly sought-after consultant in the financial services industry, and David, age 45, is a scientist who works for a major research university. Married in 1990, they had a true postmodern marriage: Both Barbara and David had high-powered careers and were committed to a role-sharing marriage. The couple graciously gave their consent to having their therapy described in this chapter, in which their identities have been disguised, and they have reviewed and commented on an earlier draft of the chapter.

The normative developmental stress of a first child transformed this role-sharing couple into a traditional marriage (see Silverstein, 1996, for a fuller description of this normative transformation). A baby, Jason, was born in November 1994. Barbara had originally planned to return to work full-time; however, after the baby was born, she panicked, feeling that she could not "abandon" Jason. She fired her childcare helper and drastically cut back on the amount of time she spent at work in order to care for Jason. Barbara described this decision as "falling on her sword" in her career.

David, in contrast, remained in his demanding job. He made some accommodations to Jason's arrival, cutting back from 100 to 60 hours per week. However, his job required that he be away often and for long stretches of time, traveling to major cities in the United States and Europe. His efforts to cut back have not been enough for Barbara, who feels utterly abandoned when he travels. His decision to take an extended series of trips when Jason was 6 weeks old hurt her "beyond the ability of words to convey." As a result, at the time therapy began, and for about a year afterward, Barbara was episodically furious at David. David, in response, felt very guilty and extremely anxious. The crisis intensified, and they entered couples therapy when Jason was 4 months old. At the beginning of therapy, the couple was clearly at an impasse. For example, at one of the first meetings Barbara said that she wanted David to be her partner. David responded that when he tries to be her partner, either in the form of suggesting plans, taking Jason, or talking to her about her life, she balks. Her rebuttal: His suggestions of plans irk her because they sound like he wants to escape from the responsibilities of parenthood, and that is the last thing she wants to hear because she feels so trapped; when he takes Jason he isn't sufficiently sensitive; and she is so furious with him she cannot talk to him about her life. As of this writing, I had seen the couple for 40 sessions over a 14-month period.

Phase 1: Learning to "Think Gender": Learning Not to Take Things Personally

From our perspective, this couple is experiencing a postmodern dilemma. They are part of the first generation to come of age in the postfeminist era. They were raised to expect that men and women can both have high-powered careers and assume equal responsibility for nurturing children.

However, traditional gender role norms remain strong in our culture. Thus, although Barbara had consciously planned to combine career and motherhood, her unexamined gut-level assumptions (resulting from her own socialization into traditional motherhood ideology) were that becoming a working mother would be the equivalent of "abandoning" her baby. Similarly, David had good intentions in terms of becoming a nurturing father. However, he became overwhelmed by his unexamined gut-level assumptions (resulting from his own socialization into traditional fatherhood ideology), which defined a good father as a "good provider." His anxiety about being able to provide adequate material resources for his family made it impossible for him to make significant changes in his commitment to work.

The first phase of work with this couple involved reframing their sense of personal betrayal and emotional abandonment as a "gender-based disappointment." Their behaviors were defined as a reversion to stereotyped gender roles, with Barbara becoming a full-time homemaker and David becoming the sole provider. Barbara did not realize that it was her own internalization of traditional mothering ideology that led her to believe that, when push comes to shove, family responsibilities fall to the woman. Rather, she felt that she was forced to sacrifice her career because David could not or would not make a commitment to sharing childcare on an equal basis. Similarly, David did not realize that his internalized vision of father as provider did not allow him to make a significant commitment to direct childcare. Rather, he felt that Barbara did not appreciate his authentic attempts to assume half of the childcare responsibilities.

It is not uncommon in states of high anxiety for people to regress to over-learned roles – in this case, those learned through traditional gender role socialization. However, most people do not realize that the birth of a child, in addition to being a positive developmental phase, is also a stressful event that generates anxiety in everyone. Without this perspective, each member of a couple often feels emotionally abandoned by his or her spouse. Learning to "think gender" helps to defuse some of the anger toward the Other.

Treating Normative Male Alexithymia (and Normative Female Emotional Flooding)

At the beginning of therapy, David was literally shaking with anxiety in the session but had great difficulty identifying his emotions and putting them into words. He had been sleeping poorly and had lost 14 lbs. Barbara, in contrast, was flooded with emotions, particularly rage and fear of abandonment, and was fighting depression.

Fortuitously Barbara was unable to make an early session due to childcare problems. This provided an opportunity to engage David in the psychoeducational program mentioned above in order to increase his emotional self-awareness. As discussed elsewhere, men often find such a structured approach with clearly defined objectives very congenial to their learning styles (Levant, 1997, 1998). David took to this work and did quite well, which helped him take responsibility for his emotions. As the work progressed over the first few months, Barbara became better able to contain her emotions and deal with them constructively, even though we were not focusing on her directly. Her progress was due in part to the fact that she felt comforted and relieved by the focus on David. His work in therapy relieved her of the responsibility of managing his emotional life as well as her own. David's increasing ability to discuss his emotions enabled him to take an active role in the problem-solving process. His increasing activity helped her to manage her anxiety so that she was then able to begin to approach him with less emotional intensity. This is a good example of how working with one member of a couple can help the other member to change as well.

Addressing the Pursuit–Distance Dynamic

Prior to these improvements, Barbara and David's impasse was a classical gender-based "pursuit–distance" (Fogarty, 1979) or "demand–withdraw" (Christensen & Heavey, 1990) relationship. Barbara became overwhelmed with her emotions, that is, her sense of isolation and anxiety about mothering. She then pursued David, pouring out her feelings and demanding that he respond and comfort her with a sense of closeness. Unfortunately, David could respond only with distancing and withdrawal, which in turn increased Barbara's sense of desperation.

David felt terribly guilty about Barbara's unhappiness. However, because of his alexithymia he was helpless in the face of her demands for empathy. He thus withdrew emotionally.

In an unconscious distancing maneuver, he often caved in to her demands about sharing childcare arrangements without fully considering their consequences in terms of his need to modify work commitments. He then did not make the necessary arrangements at work (which, in turn, was abetted by his difficulty in disappointing his colleagues) and ended up not meeting his commitments to Barbara, who felt doubly betrayed. Her despair about her situation was exacerbated by her rage at his inability to respond. She then became flooded with reactivity again, and the cycle would begin anew.

To help the couple emerge from this pursuit-distance impasse and improve their ability to resolve conflict, I taught them the standard marital communication and conflict resolution skills (empathic listening, nonreactive responding using "I" statements, and attempting to find solutions to conflicts that maximized both of their interests). They were able to use this method both in the session and at home and were moderately successful.

Initial Resolution of Reversion to Stereotyped Roles

As David's ability to identify and discuss his feelings improved, he was able to say that he was getting mixed messages from Barbara that confused and frustrated him. On the one hand, Barbara said that she wanted him to participate more in caring for Jason. However, she also had trouble relinquishing control. Sometimes he felt shut out when she was nursing or putting the baby to sleep. At other times, she was critical of his way of managing Jason.

This is another typical gender-based conflict. In the traditional family, one of the only areas in which women have had power was in terms of child rearing. Thus, although they have felt burdened by childcare, it has also been a source of power for them. Because Barbara had drastically cut back her job, childcare had now become one of the few areas in which she had power and control.

From David's perspective, traditional masculine gender role socialization had not provided him with the skills for nurturing. Although he wanted to be an active caregiver, his sense of incompetence made him particularly sensitive to Barbara's criticism. This sensitivity predisposed him to withdraw from childcare opportunities, leaving Barbara feeling abandoned. Again, gender socialization, rather than a lack of caring, was constructing their conflict.

After four months of therapy in which they were helped to understand much of their conflict as gender-based, Barbara and David were able to negotiate a shared parenting arrangement. David was to care for Jason for three-hour periods, allowing Barbara to have that time to do some professional work. Later in therapy the couple achieved a deeper and more significant resolution of this issue, which we discuss after considering the work that the couple did in Phases 2 and 3.

Phase 2: Systems-Level Change

By helping David focus on his emotional experiences, I helped him begin to take responsibility for his feelings. Through this change, he reduced the amount of Self that he was borrowing from Barbara. Similarly, I helped Barbara realize her part in their failed negotiations. Barbara was able to gain better control of her emotions and to feel less desperate. As her anxiety decreased, she had less need to pursue David in a demanding and blaming way, and he, reciprocally, felt less pressure to distance. Amelioration of the pursuing–distancing impasse allowed the couple to achieve a greater sense of closeness. From this position of greater intimacy, they were able to negotiate an arrangement that met both of their needs.

Understanding the reciprocal nature of their interaction helped each member of the couple begin to focus on the Self rather than blaming the Other. Barbara was able to understand that a part of her assuming sole responsibility for Jason emerged from her own definition of mothering, not simply because of David's failure to co-parent more equitably. David was able to articulate his definition of father as provider, which helped him understand his reluctance to limit his commitment to paid work. This realization helped him become more responsible in following through on his commitments to Barbara.

Phase 3: Family-of-Origin Issues

As the couple continued to make progress in "shifting their gaze" from Other to Self, the treatment shifted to family-of-origin issues, based on Bowen's approach of encouraging clients to rework original family relationships by practicing being a Self in the context of the family of origin.

Barbara is especially sensitive to abandonment. Her mother abandoned her to alcoholism, as she had been abandoned by her mother (Barbara's grandmother) to drug addiction. Barbara's father was a womanizer who had many affairs that were poorly hidden, including one with a maid who lived in the house. Barbara's brother is chronically depressed, and she has had bouts of depression herself. If she perceives even a subtle suggestion that Jason might be left alone, she is filled with images of the emptiness she sees in herself and her brother, and she reacts intensely. When David is gone on a business trip, she reexperiences the trauma of the early abandonment. Her attempt at mastering this trauma is to apply very high standards to caring for Jason. This need to protect Jason from her sense of abandonment is part of the reason that she finds childcare so burdensome.

In her relationship with her mother, Barbara learned to keep her feelings to herself, out of fear that if she were to say how unhappy she was she might lose her mother completely. This trait carried over to her relationship with David. She has difficulty asking directly for what she wants. She often keeps her feelings to herself, until she becomes emotionally flooded and the emotions spill out in a torrent of anger. This tendency not to share her feelings with David was abetted by David's need to distance himself from his own feelings. David's decision to travel when Jason was 6 weeks old was an example of his way of coping with his anxiety about new fatherhood. This decision was actually quite traumatic for Barbara, because she was abandoned at a time of high stress and anxiety. Subsequently, when the issue of David's travel came up she automatically assumed that he was going to abandon her and in that state of mind found it impossible to ask him for what she needed.

As therapy progressed, I made several suggestions for Barbara's family-of-origin work. After six months of therapy her mother came for a visit, and I suggested that Barbara work on trying not to lose her own voice (as is her custom with her mother) but rather try to be authentic, if only to herself. This helped her deal with her very complex set of feelings as her mother consumed alcohol on a steady basis during the visit. Working on being more authentic with her mother helped her in her relationship with David. She was able to move from assuming that he was going to abandon her, and getting furious, to being better able to calmly tell him what she needed. She thus shifted from a reactive aggressive mode to a more proactive-assertive one. I also suggested that Barbara talk with her mother about her mother's experiences with her own mother growing up. To my knowledge this has not yet happened. As it now stands, Barbara sees her mother twice a year.

At the beginning David was out of touch with his issues regarding his family. As therapy progressed, David showed an increasing capacity to look at his family-of-origin issues. Early on, the couple discussed a conflict about keeping old magazines around. To Barbara, who wanted to get rid of them, they represented "death, decay," – that is, her mother's neglect. To David, they represented his mother's intrusiveness; for example, her getting rid of a collection of scientific magazines that he had cherished.

After a couple of months of therapy David began to experience sadness when he talked about his parents. He verbalized that he was sad because he felt that they had not made the most of their lives. In one session he commented that if his father had taken a job in management (rather than the blue-collar work that he did) he would not have been injured in late midlife, and his parents might have had a better life. Similarly, after six months of therapy David was able to acknowledge that his mother's attempts to get close to him made him uncomfortable, so that has tended to keep her at a distance, much as he has done with his wife. A few sessions later he said to Barbara: "I have one for you. Don't ask me about my day. My mother used to do that, and it bugs the hell out of me." Exploring his reaction in the session, David could begin to see that more was at work than the fact that both his mother and his wife shared this "annoying trait." He began to realize that maybe if he could learn how to deal with his mother, he might not have this problem with his wife.

Phase 1 Revisited: Fuller Resolution of Gender Role Strain

Letter-Writing Exercise

After ten months of therapy David had learned to be pretty articulate about his emotions. Barbara had improved her ability to hold onto her voice and to stay her tendency to assume the worst. She was better able to ask for what she needed calmly. Yet the couple remained at an impasse. It seemed to me that the impasse was being held in place by unresolved issues resulting from events in the first six weeks of their life as parents.

Hence, I suggested that they each write a letter to the other, to be shared in the session, wherein each expressed their own experiences in those first few weeks.

This exercise was designed both to help each of them focus on the Self by examining their unique experiences and to enable them to define the Self to each other. David was surprised to learn that Barbara's bottom line commitment was to Jason, not to her career. It was important to Barbara to articulate this definition of Self, even though she had also emphasized that she felt it was unfair that she had sacrificed her career whereas David was able to continue in his work. Barbara was surprised to learn about David's feelings about the importance of the provider role. He acknowledged that he had dealt with his anxiety and feelings of inadequacy as a father by digging down and coming up with his own father's model: Be a good provider and "put a cocoon around the family." He also revealed that his antagonism toward a particular childcare provider had to do with his feelings about the fact that her salary, if pro-rated to full-time, would equal his take-home pay. Somehow, he felt that this financial arrangement trivialized his contribution to the family.

David's Growing Attachment to Jason

David began providing regular childcare for Jason in the fourth month of therapy. Barbara soon felt quite comfortable with David's parenting abilities. As a direct result of this increased and regular contact, David became completely smitten with his son.

Rebalancing the Ledger Through a Structural Change

Although the letter-writing exercise was helpful in reducing some of Barbara's smoldering antagonism and David's anxiety, the couple still remained at an impasse. It was not enough to revisit the painful period of their lives as new parents in order to find understanding and reconciliation because the basic structure of their lives still remained unworkable from Barbara's point of view. This point was driven home after about a year of therapy when David took a long series of business trips. His absence caused all of the old issues to resurface.

In one session David seemed finally to hear what Barbara had so desperately been trying to tell him: that if he wanted to hold onto his marriage, he simply had to give it a much higher priority. She made it clear that she was not going to stay in the marriage if he did not give it a higher priority.

This brought several things to a head. David had said earlier that he did not want to change his job just yet because he wanted to see things he had worked on for 20 years come to fruition. However, in response to Barbara's ultimatum, he backed down from this position, acknowledging that he has such a good record that he could do nothing for the next five years and it would not hurt his professional standing. In addition, he had by this time made some progress in overcoming his fear of being direct with colleagues. Previously he could not tell them what he felt they did not want to hear – a behavior pattern that had resulted in his failing to meet some of his commitments to Barbara. Finally, as noted above, he had fallen in love with Jason. In response to these new factors – Barbara's ability to find her voice and state her position forcefully, David's ability to state his position more directly, and David's positive attachment to Jason – David announced that he had decided to reorganize his position so as to drastically reduce both the travel and the time demands. This would free him up to share the childcare more equally with Barbara. At first Barbara was skeptical about David's commitment but a few weeks later came to feel that a corner had been turned. The quality of their interaction in the last few sessions has been decidedly more relaxed and lighthearted, as if they have both gotten through a terrible ordeal.

This therapeutic event is extremely important for the treatment of postmodern couples. In past historical periods only men had the privilege of having high-powered careers and children. In the postfeminist era women have come to expect to enjoy the same privileges. However, the birth of the first child often stimulates a regression to a traditional gender-based division of labor. When this happens, both members of the couple experience stress, as documented by Arlie Hochschild (1989), who found that conflict over sharing family responsibilities was the most common source of marital discord among dual-earner couples.

Not all couples achieve this level of structural change. Most frequently, the impetus for change comes from the wife, as it did in Barbara's case. Now that women have the potential to provide for themselves and their children, some feel entitled to demand a more equitable sharing of childcare and household responsibilities. However, traditional gender role norms are difficult to change, and many women do not find their voices on this issue. We believe that our emphasis on focusing on and defining the Self enhances the probability that both women and men will negotiate more successfully for the reciprocal benefits that postmodern marriage has to offer. Furthermore, we feel that without a serious attempt to find a more equitable gender role division of labor, resentments will continue to fester and eventually emerge as marital conflict.

Termination

I (RL) had taken a job that requires relocation out of state. This has imposed a time limit on the treatment of this case. Although the couple has made significant progress in resolving their marital impasse, work still remains to be done. Both members need to do more family-of-origin work. David needs to become better acquainted with how his family of origin has shaped his life and affected how he has functioned in his marriage. Barbara needs to continue her work on decreasing the emotional cut-off from her mother. The couple has agreed to continue their work with another family psychologist in order to maintain and consolidate their progress.

CONCLUSION

This chapter illustrates the integrated family systems-gender-based psychotherapy approach under construction by Levant and Silverstein (1996), with its multiphasic approach encompassing learning to think gender, learning to think systems, and family-of-origin work. In this chapter we paid specific attention to resolving both gender role strain and emotional fusion as co-factors in this couple's marital impasse. With regard to gender role strain, David improved his ability to be aware of and express his emotions, and Barbara was able to let go of, to some extent, the responsibilities for managing the emotional life of the couple. As David assumed more responsibility for his end, Barbara felt less emotionally flooded. With these gains under their belts, they negotiated conditions for David to provide significant blocks of child care, thereby giving Barbara time to attend to her professional responsibilities and providing David opportunities to get to know (and fall in love with) his son. The most consequential change occurred near the end of therapy, when David decided to restructure his job so that he would travel less and spend more time with Jason.

With regard to resolving the emotional fusion, the first change was seen when David improved his ability to express his own emotions, thereby changing the overall emotional system of the couple and reducing the level of conflict. The next set of changes involved Barbara making some headway in being authentic with her mother, which helped her be more proactively assertive with David, and with David confronting his fears of letting his colleagues down.

I (RL) consider it a privilege to have been able to work with David and Barbara. I learned a great deal from working with them about being a couple in the postmodern era, about resolving relationship impasses, and about integrating feminist and family systems ideas.

NOTE

1. Chapter 11, entire chapter. Copyright © 2001 by the American Psychological Association. Adapted with permission. The official citation that should be used in referencing this material is Levant, R. F., & Silverstein, L. (2001). Integrating gender and family systems theories: The "both/and" approach to treating a postmodern couple. In D. Lusterman, S. McDaniel, & C. Philpot (Eds.), *Casebook for integrating family therapy* (pp. 245–252). Washington, DC: American Psychological Association. No further reproduction or distribution is permitted without written permission from the American Psychological Association.

REFERENCES

Bowen, M. (1978). *Family therapy in clinical practice*. New York: Aronson.

Christensen, A., & Heavey, C. (1990). Gender and social structure in the demand/withdraw pattern of marital conflict. *Journal of Personality and Social Psychology*, *59*, 73–81. https://doi.org/10.1037/0022-3514.59.1.73

Fogarty, T. F (1979). The distancer and the pursuer. *The Family, 7*(1), 11–16.

Goldner, V (1988, March/April). Making room for both/and. *The Family Therapy Networker,* 55–61.

Hochschild, A. (1989). *The second shift.* New York: Viking.

Kerr, M. E., & Bowen, M. (1988). *Family evaluation.* New York: Norton.

Levant, R. F (1997). *Men and emotions: A psychoeducational approach* [Video]. Hicksville, NY: Newbridge Professional Programs. [Out of print but available from Ronald F Levant.]

Levant, R. F. (1998). Desperately seeking language: Understanding, assessing and treating normative male alexithymia. In W. Pollack & R. Levant (Eds.), *New psychotherapy for men* (pp. 35–56). New York: Wiley.

Levant, R. F., & Kopecky, G. (1995/1996). *Masculinity reconstructed: Changing the rules of manhood.* New York: Dutton/Plume. [Out of print but available from Ronald F Levant.]

Levant, R. F., & Pollack, W. S. (Eds.). (1995). *A new psychology of men.* New York: Basic Bocks.

Levant, R. F., & Silverstein, L. (1996, August). *Bridging the gap from Mars to Venus: Treating couples' impasses.* Symposium conducted at the 104th Annual Convention of the American Psychological Association, Toronto, Ontario, Canada.

Levant, R. F., & Silverstein, L. B. (2001). Integrating gender and family systems theories: The "both/and" approach to treating a postmodern couple. In S. H. McDaniel, D.-D. Lusterman, & C. L. Philpot (Eds.), *Casebook for integrating family therapy: An ecosystemic approach* (pp. 245–252). Washington, DC: American Psychological Association. https://doi-org.ezproxy.uakron.edu:2443/10.1037 /10395-019

Silverstein, L. B. (1996). Fathering is a feminist issue. *Psychology of Women Quarterly, 20,* 3–37. https://doi.org/10.1111/j.1471-6402.1996.tb00663.x

Index

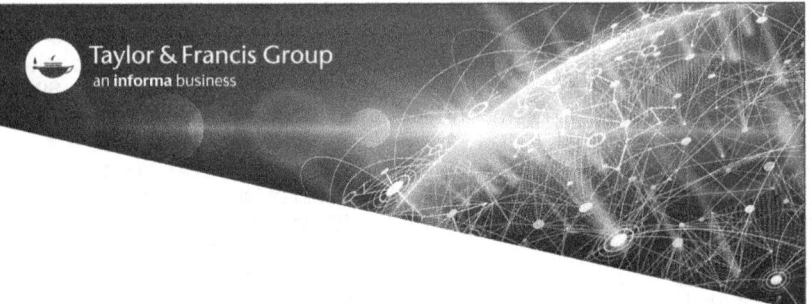
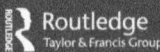
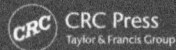